Addressing Contemporary Issues in Women's Health

Editors

STEPHANIE DEVANE-JOHNSON
JACQUELYN MCMILLIAN-BOHLER

NURSING CLINICS
OF NORTH AMERICA

www.nursing.theclinics.com

Consulting Editor
BENJAMIN SMALLHEER

December 2024 • Volume 59 • Number 4

ELSEVIER

1600 John F. Kennedy Boulevard • Suite 1800 • Philadelphia, Pennsylvania, 19103-2899

http://www.theclinics.com

NURSING CLINICS OF NORTH AMERICA Volume 59, Number 4
December 2024 ISSN 0029-6465, ISBN-13: 978-0-443-29344-3

Editor: Kerry Holland
Developmental Editor: Malvika Shah

Nursing Clinics of North America (ISSN 0029-6465) is published quarterly by Elsevier Inc., 360 Park Avenue South, New York, NY 10010-1710. Months of issue are March, June, September, and December. Periodicals postage paid at New York, NY and additional mailing offices. Subscription price per year is, $168.00 (US individuals), $275.00 (international individuals), $231.00 (Canadian individuals), $100.00 (US and Canadian students), and $135.00 (international students). For institutional access pricing please contact Customer Service via the contact information below. To receive student/resident rate, orders must be accompanied by name of affiliated institution, date of term, and the signature of program/residency coordinator on institution letterhead. Orders will be billed at individual rate until proof of status is received. Foreign air speed delivery is included in all *Clinics* subscription prices. All prices are subject to change without notice. Orders, claims, and journal inquiries: Please visit our Support Hub page https://service.elsevier.com for assistance.

Nursing Clinics of North America is covered in *EMBASE/Excerpta Medica, MEDLINE/PubMed (Index Medicus), Social Sciences Citation Index, Current Contents, ASCA, Cumulative Index to Nursing, RNdex Top 100,* and Allied Health Literature and International Nursing Index (INI).

Contributors

CONSULTING EDITOR

BENJAMIN SMALLHEER, PhD, RN, ACNP-BC, FNP-BC, CCRN, CNE, FAANP
Assistant Dean, Master of Science in Nursing Program, Associate Professor, Duke University School of Nursing, Durham, North Carolina

EDITORS

STEPHANIE DEVANE-JOHNSON, PhD, CNM, FACNM
Associate Professor, Department of Nursing, Vanderbilt University School of Nursing, Center for Research Development and Scholarship, Vanderbilt University, Nashville, Tennessee

JACQUELYN McMILLIAN-BOHLER, PhD, CNM, CNE
Assistant Professor, Department of Nursing, Duke University School of Nursing, Durham, North Carolina

AUTHORS

JESSICA AYTCH, BSW, IBCLC
Lactation Clinic Coordinator, Department of Family and Consumer Sciences, North Carolina Agricultural and Technical State University, Greensboro, North Carolina

HENRY BOHLER Jr, MD, MSc
Physician, Board Certified in Weight Management, Prospect, Kentucky

JORDON D. BOSSE, PhD, RN
Assistant Professor, College of Nursing, The University of Rhode Island, Providence, Rhode Island

EMMA BURRESS, MPH, IBCLC
Clinical Coordinator, Pathway 2 Human Lactation Training Program, North Carolina Agricultural and Technical State University, Greensboro, North Carolina

ETHAN C. CICERO, PhD, RN
Assistant Professor, tenure track, Nell Hodgson Woodruff School of Nursing, Emory University, Atlanta, Georgia

KATHERINE CROFT, BSN, RN
Program Manager, UNC Health Transgender Health Program, University of North Carolina Medical Center, Chapel Hill, North Carolina

SHIVON LATICE DANIELS, MSN, APRN, FNP-C
Nurse Practitioner, Department of Medicine, Division of Endocrinology, Metabolism, and Nutrition, Duke Heath Integrative Practice, Duke University Health System, Durham, North Carolina

STEPHANIE DEVANE-JOHNSON, PhD, CNM, FACNM
Associate Professor, Department of Nursing, Vanderbilt University School of Nursing, Center for Research Development and Scholarship, Vanderbilt University, Nashville, Tennessee

JESS DILLARD-WRIGHT, PhD, MA, RN, CNM
Associate Professor and Associate Dean of Equity and Inclusion, Elaine Marieb College of Nursing, University of Massachusetts Amherst, Amherst, Massachusetts

KELSEY FREY, MPAS, PA-C
Advanced Practice Provider, Division of Endocrinology, Duke University, Durham, North Carolina

ANGELIKA GABRIELSKI, MSN, FNP-C, APRN
Advanced Practice Provider, Division of Endocrinology, Metabolism and Nutrition, Duke University, Durham, North Carolina

ETOI GARRISON, MD
Associate Professor, Department of Obstetrics and Gynecology, Vanderbilt University Medical Center, Nashville, Tennessee

STEPHANIE GEDZYK-NIEMAN, DNP, RNC-MNN
Assistant Professor, Department of Nursing, Duke University School of Nursing, Durham, North Carolina

TANEISHA GILLYARD, PhD
Assistant Professor, Department of Biomedical Sciences, Meharry Medical College, Nashville, Tennessee

CHERYL GISCOMBE, PhD, RN, PMHNP-BC, FAAN
Interim Senior Associate Dean, Office of Academic Affairs, LeVine Family Distinguished Term Professor of Quality of Life, Health Promotion, and Wellness, UNC Chapel Hill School of Nursing, Secondary Faculty Appointment (Professor), Department of Social Medicine, School of Medicine, Chapel Hill, North Carolina

DERRICK C. GLYMPH, PhD, DNAP, CRNA, CHSE, CNE, COL, USAR, FAANA, FAAN
Associate Professor, Duke University School of Nursing, Nurse Anesthesia Program, Durham, North Carolina

BRADI GRANGER, PhD, RN, FAHA, FAAN
Professor, Duke University School of Nursing, Director, Heart Center Nursing Research Program, Duke University Health System, Duke-Margolis Center for Health Policy, Durham, North Carolina

QUINNETTE JONES, MSW, MHS, PA-C
Associate Professor, Department of Family Medicine and Community Health, Division of PA Studies, Duke University, Durham, North Carolina

BONNIE JONES-HEPLER, PhD, MSW, MSPH, RN
Assistant Professor, Duke University School of Nursing, Durham, North Carolina

MELISSA KATELLA, MSN, RN, CNE
Clinical Instructor, Duke University Health System, Durham, North Carolina

DANIEL D. KING, DNP, MNA, CRNA, APRN, CPPS, CNE
Faculty in Doctor of Nursing Practice, Nurse Anesthesia Program, Rosalind Franklin University of Medicine and Science, College of Nursing, North Chicago, Illinois

ANICA LAND, MSN, AGNP-C, APRN
Advanced Practice Provider, Division of Endocrinology, Duke University, Durham, North Carolina

ROLANDA L. LISTER, MD
Assistant Professor, Department of Obstetrics and Gynecology, Vanderbilt University Medical Center, Nashville, Tennessee

JACQUELYN McMILLIAN-BOHLER, PhD, CNM, CNE
Assistant Professor, Department of Nursing, Duke University School of Nursing, Durham, North Carolina

KRISTIN MEJIA, BA, CLC
Founder and CEO, Homeland Heart Birth and Wellness Collective, Nashville, Tennessee

JACQUETTA WOODS MELVIN, MPH, PA-C
Medical Instructor, Department of Family Medicine and Community Health, Division of Physician Assistant Studies, Duke University, Durham, North Carolina

MULUBRHAN F. MOGOS, PhD, MSc, FAHA
Assistant Professor, Department of Nursing, Vanderbilt University School of Nursing, Center for Research Development and Scholarship, Vanderbilt University, Nashville, Tennessee

AMNAZO MUHIRWA, PhD, MSN, FNP-C, BSN, RN
Postdoctoral Research Fellow, Department of Physical Medicine and Rehabilitation, Program on Integrative Medicine, University of North Carolina School of Medicine, Chapel Hill, North Carolina

DEVON NOONAN, PhD, MPH, FNP-BC, CARN, FIAAN
Dorothy L Powell Term Chair of Nursing, Associate Professor, Duke School of Nursing, Member, Duke Cancer Institute, Cancer Control and Population Sciences, Co-Director, Duke National Clinician Scholars Program, Durham, North Carolina

TAMAR RODNEY, PhD, RN, PMHNP-BC, CNE, FAAN
Assistant Professor, Johns Hopkins University School of Nursing, Baltimore, Maryland

CHRISTINE RODRIGUEZ, DNP, APRN, FNP-BC, MDIV, MA
Assistant Professor and Assistant Dean of Simulation and Clinical Innovation, Yale School of Nursing, Yale University, Orange, Connecticut

SUSAN SILVA, PhD
Associate Research Professor, Duke University School of Nursing, Durham, North Carolina

MELAN JAVONNE SMITH-FRANCIS, DNP, CNM, FNP-c
Assistant Professor, Midwifery, Bethel University, St Paul, Minnesota

VENUS STANDARD, MSN, APRN, FACNM, LCCE, CD(DONA)
Assistant Professor, Department of Family Medicine, School of Medicine, University of North Carolina, Chapel Hill, Chapel Hill, North Carolina

JANIYA MITNAUL WILLIAMS, MA, IBCLC, CLC
Clinical Instructor, Department of Family and Consumer Sciences, Program Director, Pathway 2 Human Lactation Training Program, North Carolina Agricultural and Technical State University, Greensboro, North Carolina

RISHELLE Y. ZHOU, DNAP, LLB, CRNA
Assistant Professor, Nurse Anesthesia Program, VA Portland Health Care System, Oregon Health and Science University School of Nursing, Portland, Oregon

Contents

health outcomes. The review underscores the necessity for culturally relevant stress measures in clinical practice to ensure equitable health care access and outcomes for this population.

Henry Bohler Jr.

Obesity is a disease much like any other chronic disease with multiple causes. Therefore, all contributing factors should be addressed to assist in effective weight loss. Women are twice as likely to be affected, starting at puberty. Weight reduction is challenging, in part, because of metabolic adaptations and hormonal changes that favor weight regain and these changes persist for months, if not years. Creating an energy deficit is the core of effective treatment of obesity. Physical activity is especially important to maintain weight reduction. Medications have an important role in reducing food consumption, unless contraindicated.

Derrick C. Glymph, Rishelle Y. Zhou, Daniel D. King, and Tamar Rodney

Delving into the complexities of pain management in women with polysubstance use, the focus of this article is on the intersection of chronic pain and mental health. One in 5 adults in the United States experience chronic pain, with women being particularly susceptible. To address these challenges, a careful and patient-centered is crucial. To guide our approach, we utilize the nursing process to address gender-specific factors, which influence substance use disorder, such as trauma, societal stigmas, and pain management. The significance of an interdisciplinary, multimodal approach is essential to achieve effective patient outcomes for women that misuse substances.

Shivon Latice Daniels, Jacquetta Woods Melvin, and Quinnette Jones

Nurses working in a variety of settings may encounter transgender-diverse patients. It is important for nurses and all health care providers to understand and know how to care for and provide inclusive care. This article will discuss ways to provide inclusive care as well as the health maintenance for transgender-diverse patients, and gender-affirming treatment options.

Ethan C. Cicero, Jess Dillard-Wright, Katherine Croft, Christine Rodriguez, and Jordon D. Bosse

In this article, we present a case study that illustrates the nurse's obligation in applying clinical judgment in determining the applicability and appropriateness of carrying out a standing order, and how nurses can navigate institutional policies that reinforce a gender binary and heteronormative ideals of womanhood while depriving the client of their autonomy. The case study also reveals some of the challenges transgender, nonbinary, and other gender expansive people may experience when health care institutions have standing orders that are not inclusive of all gender identities.

SERIES OF RELATED INTEREST

Advances in Family Practice Nursing
www.advancesinfamilypracticenursing.com

THE CLINICS ARE AVAILABLE ONLINE!
Access your subscription at:
www.theclinics.com

Foreword

New Era in Women's Health: Innovations and Insights

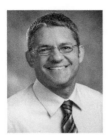

Benjamin Smallheer, PhD, RN, ACNP-BC, FNP-BC, CCRN, CNE, FAANP
Consulting Editor

In the ever-evolving landscape of medical science, the field of gender-specific health care stands as a beacon of progress and innovation. We are reminded of the profound impact advancing care for any group of individuals has, and the role research, clinical practice, and policy development has on the well-being of those individuals.

The journey of women's health has been marked by significant milestones, each contributing to a deeper understanding of the unique physiologic, psychological, and social aspects that define women's experiences. From the early days of recognizing the importance of maternal health to the contemporary focus on gender-specific medicine, the trajectory of women's health has been one of continuous growth and transformation. One of the most remarkable advancements in women's health is the interdisciplinary approach that has become the hallmark of modern research and practice. Collaboration between obstetricians, gynecologists, endocrinologists, oncologists, psychologists, and public health experts has led to groundbreaking discoveries and innovative treatments. This holistic approach ensures that women's health is addressed comprehensively, taking into account the intricate interplay of biological, environmental, and social factors.

In recent years, we have witnessed remarkable progress in several key areas of women's health. The advent of personalized medicine has revolutionized the way we approach conditions, such as breast cancer, ovarian cancer, and cardiovascular diseases. Genetic profiling and targeted therapies have not only improved survival rates but also enhanced the quality of life for countless women. In addition, advancements in reproductive health, including assisted reproductive technologies and fertility preservation, have empowered women to make informed choices about their reproductive futures. Mental health research has also gained significant attention, shedding light on the unique challenges women face, including the impact of hormonal fluctuations

Nurs Clin N Am 59 (2024) xi–xii
https://doi.org/10.1016/j.cnur.2024.09.002
0029-6465/24/© 2024 Published by Elsevier Inc.

on mood disorders and the prevalence of conditions such as postpartum depression and anxiety.

The impact of social drivers of health and the role of technology on advancing women's health cannot be overstated. Social drivers, such as socioeconomic status, education, access to health care, and cultural norms, all play a crucial role in shaping health outcomes. In addition, the implementation of technology, such as telemedicine, wearable health devices, and mobile health applications, have bridged gaps in access to care, particularly in underserved communities. Policy changes, community engagement, and advocacy are the cornerstone to creating a more equitable health care system that benefits all women, regardless of their background.

As we celebrate the achievements highlighted in this issue, we must also acknowledge the work that lies ahead. The field of women's health is dynamic, and new challenges will continue to emerge. It is our collective responsibility to remain vigilant, curious, and dedicated to advancing knowledge and practice. By fostering a culture of collaboration, innovation, and compassion, we can ensure that the future of women's health is bright and promising.

This issue of *Nursing Clinics of North America* reflects on our commitment to the health and well-being of women everywhere. Each article is dedicated to the advancements in women's health and serves as a testament to the relentless pursuit of knowledge needed to bring together a diverse array of topics, each contributing to the overarching goal of improving health outcomes for women across various stages of life and health conditions.

Benjamin Smallheer, PhD, RN, ACNP-BC, FNP-BC, CCRN, CNE, FAANP
Duke University School of Nursing
307 Trent Drive
Box 3322, Office 3117
Durham, NC 27710, USA

E-mail address:
benjamin.smallheer@duke.edu

Preface

Addressing Critical Issues in Women's Health Care

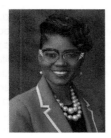
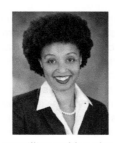

Stephanie Devane-Johnson, PhD, CNM, FACNM

Jacquelyn McMillian-Bohler, PhD, CNM, CNE

Editors

Given the dynamic nature of the women's healthcare, a comprehensive approach is essential to addressing the diverse needs and challenges faced by patients. As our understanding of these complexities grows, so must our strategies for providing inclusive, equitable, and effective care. This issue of *Nursing Clinics of North America* delves into critical areas within this field, focusing on how nurses can enhance their practice and improve patient outcomes through a thorough understanding of various topics.

Addressing birth inequity is a fundamental issue where nurses must recognize and tackle systemic and social factors contributing to disparities in maternal and neonatal health outcomes. Mitigating these inequities involves proactive interventions and advocacy to ensure equitable patient care. Parallel to addressing birth inequity, *breastfeeding support* is crucial for promoting maternal and infant health. Nurses play a pivotal role in assisting with latching techniques, managing common issues such as engorgement and nipple pain, and providing education to help establish successful breastfeeding practices. Transitioning from breastfeeding support, the *BRIDGE conceptual framework* introduces a model for integrating doula support throughout the pregnancy continuum. This framework emphasizes the importance of continuous, holistic support and guides nurses in incorporating doula practices into their care models to enhance maternal outcomes. The *fourth trimester* represents a significant, yet often overlooked, phase of postpartum care. During this period, nurses must focus on maternal recovery and infant care, addressing physical, emotional, and developmental needs. Effective management involves monitoring recovery from childbirth, providing emotional support, and guiding new parents through infant care routines.

Similarly, *complementary and alternative medicine* offers additional options for managing menopausal symptoms. Nurses need to be knowledgeable about the efficacy

https://doi.org/10.1016/j.cnur.2024.08.010
0029-6465/24/© 2024 Published by Elsevier Inc.
nursing.theclinics.com

and safety of these treatments to provide balanced recommendations. Addressing conditions such as *polycystic ovarian syndrome (PCOS)* involves understanding its impact on women's health and applying appropriate management strategies. Nurses can support patients in managing PCOS through lifestyle interventions and medical treatments. Another significant topic is the *psychometric scales of the Strong Black Woman construct*, which evaluates stress-related health disparities among African American women. Insights from these scales can help nurses better understand and address the unique challenges faced by this population. Addressing *obesity management in women* involves understanding its impact and employing effective strategies for management, including lifestyle changes and medical interventions. In the context of *polysubstance use*, a nursing process approach to pain management is crucial, offering strategies to address pain while considering the complexities of substance use. *Caring for transgender patients* requires specific knowledge and practices to ensure respectful and effective care, highlighting the need for continued education and inclusivity in nursing practice. Last, supporting *women and transfeminine clients navigating noninclusive standing orders* involves advocacy and practical support to help clients overcome barriers and ensure their needs are met.

Each of these topics represents a crucial aspect of comprehensive nursing care. Through this issue, we aim to provide valuable insights and strategies to enhance nursing practice and patient outcomes across these diverse areas. By exploring these interconnected themes, we hope to empower nurses with the knowledge and tools necessary to navigate the multifaceted challenges of modern health care. As we continue to advance our understanding of women's health, it is our collective responsibility to ensure that our practices evolve to meet the changing needs of our patients, fostering a more inclusive, equitable, and effective health care system for all.

DISCLOSURES

The guest editors have no known conflicts of interest.

Stephanie Devane-Johnson, PhD, CNM, FACNM
Vanderbilt University School of Nursing
461 21st Avenue South
Nashville, TN 37240, USA

Jacquelyn McMillian-Bohler, PhD, CNM, CNE
Duke University School of Nursing
307 Trent Drive
Durham, NC 27701, USA

E-mail addresses:
Stephanie.devane-johnson@vanderbilt.edu (S. Devane-Johnson)
Jmm234@duke.edu (J. McMillian-Bohler)

Addressing Birth Inequity
A Guide for Nurses

Jacquelyn McMillian-Bohler, PhD, CNM, CNE[a],*,
Stephanie Devane-Johnson, PhD, CNM, FACNM[b],
Venus Standard, MSN, APRN, FACNM, LCCE, CD(DONA)[c]

KEYWORDS

- Maternal mortality • Infant mortality • Birth inequity • Birth equity • Bias
- Health equity

KEY POINTS

- US maternal and infant mortality disproportionately affects underrepresented populations and are the highest among all developed counties.
- The reasons for the disparate maternal mortality disparities are multifaceted, including racism, lack of access to care, and preexisting conditions such as cardiovascular conditions, factors, obesity, and diabetes.
- Person-centered care can improve maternal and infant health outcomes, especially for underrepresented and marginalized groups.
- If nurses use bias mitigation strategies, they can provide more equitable and culturally intelligent care to birthing persons, infants, and their families.

INTRODUCTION

Maternal mortality represents the death of a person during pregnancy or within 42 days of termination of pregnancy from causes related to or worsened by the pregnancy or care received during pregnancy.[1] In 2022, the maternal mortality rate in the United States was 22.3 deaths per 100,000 live births.[1] Although this rate is a significant decrease from 32.9 in 2021, the United States continues to experience the highest maternal and infant mortality rates among developed countries.[2] A closer review of the maternal mortality data reveals significant disparities in outcomes by ethnicity, socioeconomic status, and age. Black women experience a maternal mortality rate of 49.5 deaths per 100,000 live births, which is significantly higher than the rates for White (19.0), Hispanic (16.9), and Asian (13.2) women. Women under the age of 25

[a] Department of Nursing, Duke University School of Nursing, 307 Trent Drive, Durham, NC 27710, USA; [b] Department of Nursing, Vanderbilt University School of Nursing, Nashville, TN 37240, USA; [c] Department of Family Medicine, University of North Carolina at Chapel Hill, 590 Manning Drive, Chapel Hill, NC 27514, USA
* Corresponding author.
E-mail address: Jmm234@duke.edu

Nurs Clin N Am 59 (2024) 511–518
https://doi.org/10.1016/j.cnur.2024.09.001   **nursing.theclinics.com**

experience death during pregnancy at the rate of 20.1 per 100,000 births, 31.3 for women 25-39.[1] And women over 40 138 deaths per 100,000 births. Birthing persons living in rural areas experience double the mortality rate than those living in urban areas.[3] The reasons behind these disparities are multifaceted, including racism, lack of access to care, and preexisting conditions such as cardiovascular conditions, factors, obesity, and diabetes.[4] According to the Center for Disease Control, however, 84% of the deaths are preventable.[1]

Infant mortality refers to the death of an infant before their first birthday.[5] The infant mortality rate is the number of infant deaths for every 1,000 live births, and along with maternal mortality serves as a crucial marker of a society's overall health.[6] Between 2019 and 2021, the average infant mortality rate per 1,000 live births in the United States was highest among Black infants at 10.5, followed by American Indian/Alaska Native infants at 5.3, Hispanic infants at 4.8, White infants at 4.4, and Asian/Pacific Islander infants at 3.6.[5] Black infants are twice as likely to die before their first birthday compared to their White peers, with the primary causes of infant deaths being prematurity and low birth weight.[7] Non-Hispanic Black/African American infants are almost 4 times as likely to die from complications related to low birthweight as compared to non-Hispanic White infants. Additionally, in 2020, non-Hispanic Black/African American infants had 2.9 times the deaths from sudden infant death syndrome as non-Hispanic Whites.[7] These statistics highlight significant health disparities and underscore the need for continued efforts to address these inequities.

Prioritizing person-centered care can enhance maternal and infant health outcomes, particularly for underrepresented and marginalized groups. The American Nurse Association Code of Ethics[8] mandates that nurses provide fair and equitable clinical care. Nurses must ensure equitable childbirth treatment for all patients. To achieve equity in obstetric care, nurses need to understand maternal and infant mortality rates, recognize biases, and work to reduce them. Understanding the differences between equity, equality, justice, and inclusion is vital for delivering quality, individualized care that meets each patient's unique needs. This article aims to offer a resource on equitable care principles and bias mitigation strategies in obstetric care. Understanding equitable care requires understanding of the definitions of several terms: equity, equality, justice, and inclusion, which will be presented next.

THE FOUNDATION OF PROVIDING EQUITABLE CARE
Definitions

Differentiating between equity and equality is a crucial step in providing equitable care. Equality ensures that everyone receives the same resources.[9] While this approach seems fair, it does not focus on outcomes or guarantee quality care for everyone. For example, ensuring that everyone receives the same number of prenatal visits and prenatal vitamins and has a hospital nearby achieves equality. However, a high-risk client may require more frequent visits, or a client with a demanding work schedule may need help to make scheduled visits during working hours. Even if the resources are the same for all (ie, equal), the outcomes will differ for these patients.

Equity ensures everyone receives the necessary resources to achieve similar outcomes.[9] Equity is not a one-size-fits-all approach; the resources are tailored and distributed based on each client's unique needs. To provide this type of individualized care, one must possess a genuine interest in understanding the experiences of people who have a different life experience. Care cannot be individualized without knowing what someone needs. Justice, like equity, ensures individuals receive what they deserve. Reproductive justice further explores the concept of justice, requiring that every person should have autonomy and control over whether they have children, how they will have children, and how they will raise their children in a safe environment.[10]

Inclusion requires providing resources to everyone, especially those who may be marginalized. Respect is another important concepts in heath equity. Respect is not just a courtesy but a fundamental aspect of nursing care. It implies that we highly regard their wishes and desires, promoting their dignity and well-being.[11] Altogether, these concepts represent a set of foundational principles that should guide the nurse's interaction with all patients and clients.

Identifying and Addressing Biases

To deliver fair care, nurses need to start by acknowledging their own biases.[12] Additionally, they should commit to offering equitable care through strategies such as cultural intelligence and crafting policies and protocols that ensure fairness. The detailed strategies for each step in this process are presented later.

Becoming Aware of Biases

Bias, a fundamental aspect of human nature, influences health care decision-making and can result in disparities.[13,14] There are 2 main types: explicit bias, which we consciously recognize, and implicit bias, which operates unconsciously. While explicit bias is less prevalent in health care, implicit bias can affect areas such as maternity care, leading to variations in pain management and counseling that differ by race.[14] Tools like the Grobman tool, which incorporate racial factors, highlight these disparities. Cognitive bias pertains to decisions influenced by personal preferences, affecting how patients' needs are addressed. To combat inequities in childbirth, health care providers must be aware of and counteract their biases.

The Implicit Bias Association Test (IAT)[15,16] was introduced in 2003 to help individuals uncover their own biases. The IAT assesses the strength of associations between concepts and evaluations by measuring response times during word-sorting tasks. Over 40 million assessments have been conducted to date. Analysis of the IAT results shows that most people have biases they are unaware of, that these biases can predict behavior, and that people exhibit different levels of bias. Another strategy to increase awareness of bias is a structured self-reflection process.

A Stepwise Approach to Self-reflection

The process begins with (1) reflection, where individuals reflect on their experiences, beliefs, and attitudes toward different racial and ethnic groups. In step 2, biases are further (2) explored through expressive activities like journaling. After identifying the bias, the next step is to (3) acknowledge these biases without judgment and work to (4) understand how the biases present and impact others. In step (5), the individuals educate themselves on how the biases may have affected a group from the historical context. Based on this understanding, it is possible to (6) implement strategies to change. They then implement change (Step 6) by developing techniques such as practicing cultural intelligence and seeking feedback. Step (7) includes a continuous improvement process to monitor and respond to bias. Implementing Equitable Care Practices.

STRATEGIES FOR MITIGATING BIASES

Since the late 90s, cultural intelligence has been aimed at reducing bias in many settings. The Cultural Intelligence (CQ) Framework©,[17] emphasizing effective cross-cultural work, includes 4 components: CQ Drive, Knowledge, Strategy, and Behavior. **Table 1** shows how these elements can help reduce bias in maternity care.

Table 1
Description and application of the cultural intelligence framework©[17]

CQ Tenant	Description[17]	General Actions Consistent with the CQ Concept	CQ Applied to Caring for a Birthing Person
Drive/Motivation	The interest and confidence to adapt to multicultural situations. It involves the willingness to learn about and engage with different cultures.	Joining local and national organizations that support and advocate for women from underrepresented groups. Actively seeking out opportunities to learn about the cultural practices and beliefs of the diverse families they care for.	The Obstetrical (OB) nurse might demonstrate CQ drive by attending workshops or training sessions on cultural competence in maternal and infant care, showing a genuine interest in understanding and respecting the cultural backgrounds of their patients
Knowledge/ Cognition	This involves understanding cultural similarities and differences. It includes knowledge about cultural norms, practices, and conventions in different cultural settings.	Regularly attending educational programs and training workshops aimed at educating health professionals about racism and bias (eg, opportunities presented by experts in CQ, diversity, and inclusion seminars).	The OB nurse might learn about the traditional birthing practices and postpartum rituals of a particular cultural group and incorporate this knowledge into their care plans to ensure culturally sensitive and respectful care.
Strategy/ Metacognition	Making sense of culturally diverse experiences and planning accordingly. It involves being aware of one's own cultural assumptions and adjusting one's strategy to interact effectively in different cultural contexts.	Developing strategies to promote anti-racist practices (eg, paying attention to implicit biases, addressing macroaggressions, and creating opportunities for social interaction with diverse groups). Reflecting on their own cultural biases and developing a plan to communicate effectively with patients from diverse backgrounds.	An OB nurse might create a checklist of culturally appropriate questions to ask during patient encounters to better understand the patient's preferences and needs, ensuring that their care is tailored to each family's unique cultural context.
Behavior/Action	The ability to adapt one's behavior to different cultural contexts. It includes having a flexible range of behaviors that can be used appropriately in various cultural situations	Moving beyond planning and educational programs toward the implementation of anti-racist initiatives that improve maternal outcomes for women from underrepresented groups (eg, implementing events designed to promote anti-racism and oppose tolerance for racist language and behaviors, using translation services consistently).	An OB nurse might adapt their behavior to different cultural contexts by using appropriate communication styles and body language. For example, they might use more formal language and maintain a respectful distance when interacting with patients from cultures that value formality and personal space; or, they might learn key phrases in the patient's native language to build rapport and trust.

About Cultural Intelligence | Cultural Intelligence Center. Published October 30, 2018. Accessed August 3, 2024. https://culturalq.com/about-cultural-intelligence/.

COMMITMENT TO PROVIDING PERSON-CENTERED CARE

The World Health Organization (WHO) has set benchmarks to enhance maternal and newborn care quality. These guidelines aim to guarantee that every woman and newborn receives top-notch care during pregnancy, delivery, and the postnatal phase. The following **Table 2** is a summary of the essential standards.

ENSURING EQUITABLE CARE PROTOCOLS

The WHO[18] *also suggests* equitable care protocols in maternity care aim to ensure that all patients receive high-quality, respectful, and individualized care regardless of their background. Here are some examples.

1. *Comprehensive Care During Labor:* This involves monitoring the birthing person and fetus during the antepartum period, managing pain effectively, providing care for the neonate immediately after birth, supporting postpartum clients during the recovery period, and facilitating safe birthing experiences for both the individual and the baby
2. *Reproductive Justice Principles:* Applying knowledge of reproductive justice principles and social determinants of health to provide equitable care to diverse populations during pregnancy, labor, and postpartum periods
3. *Holistic Management of Pregnancies:* This includes care during labor, neonatal care, and support for early parenthood, emphasizing reproductive justice, social determinants of health, and family well-being
4. *Mental Health Care:* Delivering safe, equitable, culturally appropriate, evidence-based care in psychiatric and mental health nursing, including the nurse-client relationship, pharmacologic management, mental health disorders, and promoting mental wellness for a diverse population

Case Study: Equitable Care Practices in Nursing for a Birthing Person

Background

Alex, a 30-year-old birthing person, arrived at the hospital in labor. Alex's socioeconomic status was challenging; they worked a minimum-wage job and lacked comprehensive

Table 2
Summary of world health organization *Standards for Maternal and Neonatal Care*[18]

Standard	Description
Provision of Care:	Ensuring that care is provided in a timely, respectful, and non-discriminatory manner. This includes always having skilled health personnel available and providing care that is evidence-based and tailored to the needs of the mother and newborn.
Experience of Care:	Respecting the dignity, privacy, and confidentiality of women and newborns. This involves effective communication, informed decision-making, and providing emotional support to women and their families.
Availability of Resources:	Ensuring that essential medicines, equipment, and supplies are available and accessible. This includes having functional health facilities with adequate infrastructure and resources to provide quality care.
Health Information Systems:	Implementing robust health information systems to monitor and evaluate the quality of care. This involves collecting and analyzing data on maternal and newborn health outcomes to inform policy and practice.

health insurance. Additionally, Alex had limited health literacy, making it difficult to understand medical terminology and procedures. Alex also had a history of hypertension, which required careful monitoring during labor and delivery.

Challenges
Alex faced several barriers to receiving equitable care as follows

1. *Socioeconomic Status:* Limited financial resources and lack of comprehensive health insurance.
2. *Health Literacy:* Difficulty understanding medical information and instructions.
3. *Level of Wellness:* History of hypertension requiring specialized care.
4. *Bias:* Potential biases related to their socioeconomic status and health literacy.

Intervention
The nursing team at the hospital implemented several equitable care practices to address these challenges.

1. *Comprehensive Assessment:* The nursing team conducted a thorough assessment of Alex's medical history, socioeconomic status, and health literacy. This assessment helped identify her specific needs and potential barriers to care.
2. *Patient Education:* Recognizing Alex's limited health literacy, the nurses used simple language and visual aids to explain the labor and delivery process. They provided written materials in plain language and used teach-back methods to ensure Alex understood the information. The nurses also took extra time to answer any questions Alex had, ensuring she felt comfortable and informed.
3. *Care Coordination:* The nursing team collaborated with a social worker to address Alex's financial concerns. The social worker helped Alex apply for emergency Medicaid to cover her hospital expenses and connected her with community resources for postpartum support. This coordination ensured that Alex had access to necessary services without the added stress of financial burdens.
4. *Personalized Care Plan:* The nurses developed a personalized care plan that included frequent monitoring of Alex's blood pressure due to her history of hypertension. They also provided continuous labor support, including pain management options and emotional support, to ensure Alex felt comfortable and informed throughout the process. The nurses made sure to involve Alex in decision-making, respecting her preferences and choices.
5. *Cultural Sensitivity and Bias Mitigation:* The nursing team was trained in cultural competence and made a conscious effort to respect Alex's cultural background and preferences. They ensured that Alex's partner was involved in the decision-making process and provided emotional support. To mitigate bias, the nurses participated in regular training sessions on implicit bias and equitable care practices. They also used standardized protocols and checklists to ensure that all patients received the same level of care, regardless of their background or circumstances.
6. *Supportive Environment:* The nurses created a supportive and non-judgmental environment for Alex. They actively listened to Alex's concerns and validated her feelings, fostering a sense of trust and safety. The nurses also advocated for Alex's needs, ensuring that her voice was heard and respected by the entire health care team.

Outcome
Alex successfully delivered a healthy baby. The equitable care practices implemented by the nursing team ensured that Alex received comprehensive,

personalized, and culturally sensitive care. Alex expressed gratitude for the support and education she received, which empowered them to make informed decisions about their care. The collaboration with the social worker also helped alleviate Alex's financial concerns, allowing her to focus on her recovery and newborn care.

Conclusion

This case study demonstrates the importance of addressing socioeconomic status, health literacy, level of wellness, and potential biases in providing equitable care to birthing persons. By implementing comprehensive assessments, patient education, care coordination, personalized care plans, cultural sensitivity, and bias mitigation strategies, health care providers can ensure that all patients receive the care they need, regardless of their background or circumstances.

CHALLENGES AND SOLUTIONS

- *Common Challenges:*
  - Identifying and addressing barriers to implementing equitable care, such as systemic issues and resource limitations.
  - Overcoming resistance to change and fostering a culture of equity.
- *Solutions:*
  - *Collaborative Approaches:* Working with interdisciplinary teams to address challenges and improve care.
  - *Policy and Advocacy:* Engaging in advocacy efforts to promote equitable policies and practices at institutional and community levels.
  - *Resource Allocation:* Strategies for effective use of resources to support equitable care initiatives.

SUMMARY

The journey toward equitable maternal and child health care is both a necessary and complex endeavor. This document has highlighted the alarming disparities in birth outcomes, particularly among women of color and those in rural communities and underscored the critical need for systemic change. By understanding and implementing the principles of equitable care, addressing both explicit and implicit biases, and committing to person-centered care, we can begin to dismantle the barriers that contribute to these disparities. As we move forward, it is imperative that we continue to advocate for policies and practices that prioritize the health and well-being of all mothers and infants. Together, we can work toward a future where every birth is met with the highest standard of care and an equal chance at life.

CLINICS CARE POINTS

- Clinicians must acknowledge and address both explicit and implicit bias to provide equitable care.

- Equitable healthcare care ensures that everyone receives the necessary resources to achieve similar outcomes, which requires understanding and addressing each patient's unique needs.

- The cultural intelligence framework can be used to increase effectiveness of healthcare providers in caring for a diverse patient population.

REFERENCES

1. Hoyer. Maternal mortality rates in the United States, 2021. 2023. Available at: https://www.cdc.gov/nchs/data/hestat/maternal-mortality/2021/maternal-mortality-rates-2021.htm. Accessed August 3, 2024.
2. American Public Health Association. Reducing US maternal mortality as a human right. Reducing US maternal mortality as a human right. 2024. Available at: https://www.apha.org/policies-and-advocacy/public-health-policy-statements/policy-database/2014/07/11/15/59/reducing-us-maternal-mortality-as-a-human-right. Accessed August 3, 2024.
3. Singh GK. Trends and social inequalities in maternal mortality in the United States, 1969-2018. Int J MCH AIDS 2020;10(1):29–42.
4. Harrington KA, Cameron NA, Culler K, et al. Rural–urban disparities in adverse maternal outcomes in the United States, 2016–2019. Am J Public Health 2023; 113(2):224–7.
5. CDC. Infant mortality. Maternal infant health. 2024. Available at: https://www.cdc.gov/maternal-infant-health/infant-mortality/index.html. Accessed September 3, 2024.
6. American Journal of Managed Care. US has highest infant, Maternal Mortality Rates Despite the Most Health Care Spending. AJMC; 2023. Available at: https://www.ajmc.com/view/us-has-highest-infant-maternal-mortality-rates-despite-the-most-health-care-spending. Accessed August 3, 2024.
7. US Department of Health and Human Services. Infant mortality and African Americans | office of minority health. Available at: https://minorityhealth.hhs.gov/infant-mortality-and-african-americans. Accessed August 3, 2024.
8. Hegge M. Code of Ethics for nurses with interpretive statements. Silver Spring, MD: American Nurses Association; 2015.
9. Miller ML, Dupree J, Monette MA, et al. Health equity and perinatal mental health. Curr Psychiatr Rep 2024;26(9):460–9.
10. Bachorik AE, Shankar M, Williams M, et al. Teaching reproductive justice. Clin Teach 2023;20(4):e13593.
11. CDC. Health equity principles to develop inclusive communications. Centers for Disease Control and Prevention; 2022. Available at: https://www.cdc.gov/health communication/Comm_Dev.html. Accessed August 3, 2024.
12. Shah HS, Bohlen J. Implicit bias. In: StatPearls. StatPearls Publishing; 2024. Available at: http://www.ncbi.nlm.nih.gov/books/NBK589697/. Accessed August 3, 2024.
13. Narayan MC. CE: addressing implicit bias in nursing: a review. Am J Nurs 2019; 119(7):36–43.
14. Saluja B, Bryant Z. How implicit bias contributes to racial disparities in maternal morbidity and mortality in the United States. J Wom Health 2021;30(2):270–3.
15. Greenwald AG, McGhee DE, Schwartz JLK. Measuring individual differences in implicit cognition: the implicit association test. J Pers Soc Psychol 1998;74(6): 1464–80.
16. Impliciat bias assessment tool. Available at: https://implicit.harvard.edu/implicit/takeatest.html. Accessed August 1, 2024.
17. About cultural intelligence | cultural intelligence center. 2018. Available at: https://culturalq.com/about-cultural-intelligence/. Accessed August 3, 2024.
18. World Health Organization. Prioritizing quality of care in maternal health. Available at: https://www.who.int/activities/prioritizing-quality-of-care-in-maternal-health. Accessed August 3, 2024.

Nurturing the Journey
Preparing for Breastfeeding and Beyond

Janiya Mitnaul Williams, MA, IBCLC, CLC[a],*,
Emma Burress, MPH, IBCLC[b], Jessica Aytch, BSW, IBCLC[c],
Stephanie Devane-Johnson, PhD, CNM, FACNM[d]

KEYWORDS

- Breastfeeding • Preconception health • Prenatal education • Cultural sensitivity
- Maternal medications • Lactation support • Postpartum care
- Community empowerment

KEY POINTS

- Importance of preconception health: Highlighting the role of preconception health in preparing for pregnancy and breastfeeding.
- Cultural sensitivity in breastfeeding support: Addressing the need for culturally sensitive lactation support to overcome barriers among diverse communities.
- Maternal medications and breastfeeding: Discussing the challenges and considerations regarding medication use during breastfeeding.
- Role of support systems: Emphasizing the crucial role of support systems in facilitating successful breastfeeding journeys.
- Community empowerment for breastfeeding: Advocating for community-based initiatives to empower families and promote breastfeeding as a public health priority.

There are many things to think about in the early days of pregnancy or planning to get pregnant. Envisioning your ideal birth, the selection of your care provider, where your baby will be born and how your family plans to feed your baby are some of the principal talking points. The list is endless and can be overwhelming. One of the prime places to start is to prioritize self-care. The benefit of adopting healthy habits before pregnancy is one way to set both oneself and one's future child on a path of health

[a] Pathway 2 Human Lactation Training Program, North Carolina Agricultural & Technical State University, Benbow Hall Suite, 202-C, 1601 E. Market Street, Greensboro, NC 22411, USA; [b] Pathway 2 Human Lactation Training Program North Carolina Agricultural & Technical State University, Benbow Hall Suite 208-D, 1601 E. Market Street, Greensboro, NC 22411, USA; [c] North Carolina Agricultural & Technical State University, Benbow Hall Suite 208-D, 1601 E. Market Street, Greensboro, NC 22411, USA; [d] Department of Nursing, Vanderbilt University, 461 21st Avenue South, Nashville, TN 37240, USA
* Corresponding author.
E-mail address: jtmitnau@ncat.edu

Nurs Clin N Am 59 (2024) 519–526
https://doi.org/10.1016/j.cnur.2024.07.005
nursing.theclinics.com
0029-6465/24/© 2024 Elsevier Inc. All rights reserved, including those for text and data mining, AI training, and similar technologies.

and well-being that can have lifelong impacts.[1] The Health in Preconception, Pregnancy and Postpartum Global Alliance developed a set of 5 preconception priorities that were published in 2019:[2]

1. Healthy diet and nutrition
2. Weight management
3. Physical activity
4. Planned pregnancy including awareness and optimizing fertility
5. Physical, mental, and psychosocial health

Exploring ones' beliefs and behaviors around nutrition and exercise before one conceives is important and sets the framework to engage in conversations around recommendations with ones' chosen care provider.[3] Pregnancy is a time when there are often many barriers to healthy eating and physical activity, including potential nausea and fatigue. Initiating a proactive approach to nutritional and physical health, alongside considerations regarding exercise and personal nutrition, facilitates the ability to navigate potential barriers with care providers more effectively. Emphasizing self-care not only lays the foundation for a healthy pregnancy but also prepares for the breastfeeding journey postbirth, which imposes additional nutritional and energy requirements on the postpartum body.

When preparing to decide how to feed your baby, accessing evidence-based information from providers and self-taught resources is crucial. We hope adequate information and conversations with professionals will empower the family to make a feeding plan that works for everyone. Typically, this decision is made largely based on the desires of the parent who would be feeding the baby, but health benefits, social, financial, and religious considerations are often part of the process.[4] One element of the decision-making process is whether breastfeeding fits with the health care needs of the feeding parent.

The need for maternal medications can become a barrier to breastfeeding. This is primarily due to a lack of information and conversation on the benefits and risks of breastfeeding while using certain medications. Ultimately, parents should have thorough conversations with their care providers before stopping their medications or halting breastfeeding due to medication concerns. The US Food and Drug Administration introduced a Pregnancy and Lactation Labeling Rule in 2015. Safety information for pregnancy and lactation is now more easily accessible, but due to the limited research conducted, most often, there is little information listed.[5–7] Care providers and the general population can access more detailed information on the safety of medications for use during breastfeeding through databases like LactMed[8] and Hale's Medication and Mother's Milk.[9] A healthy parent is a very important part of the breastfeeding dyad, and lactating parents should explore all of their options for their own care to enable them to make a fully informed decision about breastfeeding while on medications.

The decision to breastfeed or chestfeed is based on the acknowledgment of the significant health advantages it provides not just to infants but also to parents themselves. However, this choice is accompanied by various obstacles, including challenges such as returning to work and dealing with pain from improper latching and positioning. Despite these hurdles, many mothers and birthing individuals initiate nursing and actively seek solutions to overcome these barriers. Finding comprehensive support, assistance, and guidance is crucial to empowering parents in their breastfeeding journey. It is important to recognize that nursing success heavily relies on support, both from health care providers and within the social network of the parent. Support plays a critical role in helping parents navigate challenges and uncertainties associated with nursing, providing encouragement, guidance, and practical assistance along the way. By fostering a supportive environment, parents are better equipped to overcome hurdles and achieve their feeding goals, ultimately promoting better health outcomes.

Breastfeeding success is profoundly influenced by a multitude of factors, among which education and information, health care access, and strong support systems stand out. Of these, the mother/birthing person's partner and family members emerge as the most influential when shaping infant feeding choice.[10] These individuals play a crucial role in facilitating the successful initiation and continuation of breastfeeding, fostering the well-being of the dyad. Studies have provided evidence showing a strong correlation between family support and maternal self-efficacy in exclusive breastfeeding/chestfeeding.[11] Nursing people with these elements are also more likely to meet their personal breastfeeding/chestfeeding goals compared to those lacking assistance.

It is also important to note that those from diverse cultural backgrounds, in particular, Black mothers and birthing people, require more than just support from family and friends but also from lactation support professionals who share similar racial backgrounds, highlighting the significance of increasing the presence of Black International Board Certified Lactation Consultants (IBCLCs).[12] Black lactation professionals are rapidly entering the field by way of mentorship and through academic programs. There are notably 2 academic programs for lactation at Historically Black Colleges and Universities; North Carolina Agricultural and Technical State University (NC A&T), and Johnson C. Smith University.[13] The primary objectives of the Lactation Program at NC A&T are to (1) increase breastfeeding/chestfeeding rates for all marginalized populations, especially Black and Brown families; (2) diversify the lactation workforce by creating more IBCLCs of color; and (3) produce more culturally aware IBCLCs.[14]

Cultural and social influences also play a significant role in shaping infant feeding decisions, once again highlighting the importance of culturally sensitive support mechanisms to ensure that all families feel empowered to make informed choices that align with their values and beliefs. A study by Devane-Johnson, revealed that "mammy" stereotypes associated with Black women and breastfeeding have also impacted infant feeding practices.[15] These stereotypes along with societal norms such as returning to work, and the early introduction to solid foods shape perceptions and behaviors related to nursing.

Recognizing the diversity in family needs and preferences, particularly regarding breastfeeding/chestfeeding and human milk feeding, is crucial. Infant feeding is not a one-size-fits-all approach, particularly when it comes to breastfeeding. It is necessary to acknowledge and educate families on the range of feeding options available including: exclusively pumping and providing their milk, combination feeding, formula feeding, and exclusive nursing. While accepting and supporting diverse feeding practices, it is important to accentuate the unparalleled advantages of human milk and offer ongoing support and infant feeding education to families.

When choosing to breastfeed/chestfeed, birthing individuals, their families, support systems, and communities require accessible and readily available resources. This is essential to ensure the delivery of respectful, culturally appropriate, nonstigmatizing, and evidence-based care, which forms the foundation for achieving their lactation goals.[16] Among these resources, prenatal lactation education stands out as paramount, laying the groundwork for informed decision-making and successful breastfeeding journeys.

The significance of breastfeeding families having comprehensive support cannot be overstated. Receiving this type of support is undeniably beneficial for nursing parents, but it also highlights the crucial role of those providing assistance in offering comprehensive education. In today's age of misinformation, finding reliable lactation information can be daunting. Early breastfeeding education plays a pivotal role in equipping parents with the knowledge and skills necessary to navigate the complexities of breastfeeding successfully.

Many local hospitals offer an array of virtual and in-person educational resources for expecting families for low or no cost. Basic breastfeeding classes acquaint families with introductory information to start them on an informed journey of lactation. Topics discussed typically include information on what to expect when their baby is born, establishing a sufficient milk supply, milk production expectations, breastfeeding positions, identifying characteristics of an effective latch and milk transfer, hunger cues, and signs of satiation to name a few. Hospital breastfeeding classes also help families learn how to request lactation assistance during their hospital stay as well as how to access outpatient lactation support. In 2017, it was reported that 98.4% of births took place in a hospital, showcasing that hospital resources are often the most accessible.[17] However, birth centers, local birth workers, and community maternal health organizations offer lactation classes and workshops to families seeking an alternative approach to lactation education. Out-of-hospital resources may also allow families to receive education from communities that may closely align with their philosophies and identities.

State and county agencies provide lactation education to expecting families within their jurisdiction. The WIC program, which stands for the special supplemental nutrition program for women, infants, and children, allocates federal grants to states for supplemental foods, health care referrals, and nutritional education. These resources are available to pregnant individuals, breastfeeding parents, nonbreastfeeding postpartum individuals, as well as infants and children up to the age of 5 years. Families that meet the income qualifications to be WIC recipients have access to breastfeeding peer counselors who provide support and basic breastfeeding education in a myriad of settings such as the WIC where parents can discuss challenges and concerns on a one-on-one basis. Many WIC offices offer breastfeeding classes and host parent-led support groups. Some WIC peer counselors call new and expectant parents to answer questions in between appointments, visit clients in the hospital to assist them with getting a good start, and make home visits to meet the needs of those who are unable to travel. Beyond the offerings that WIC provides, many counties have resource lists available online or in guidebooks that include information about programs that offer additional lactation education and support resources.[18]

In this day in age, many people obtain information from social media platforms that create access to all types of information at lightning speed. Generations are now using social media sites as search engines. With the growing popularity of social media applications, it is important to be able to identify accurate avenues of information as popular content creators are being regarded as experts. Lactation organizations and many credentialed professionals are using social media sites to create better access to pertinent information. It is important to verify the credentials of the individual disseminating the information. Credentialed lactation professionals are known as Certified Lactation Counselors (CLCs) such as breastfeeding peer counselors, IBCLCs, and other supportive health care providers. Evidence suggests that peer-to-peer lactation education is effective, however; it is important to keep in mind that one person's lactation experience is uniquely theirs, and the information that they acquired during their journey may or may not be effective for new and expecting parents.

Historically, books have consistently served as a dependable and precise source of information. Many expecting families utilize books to obtain knowledge on pertinent subject matters as their schedule permits in the comfort of the environment of their choosing. An additional advantage is that the authors commonly offer online support via forums, groups, and communities for those seeking further connection with like-minded peers as an extension of their book. The books that have been highly regarded as credible sources of information that provided helpful information and positively influenced successful lactation journeys are

1. *Feed the Baby: An Inclusive Guide to Nursing, Bottle-Feeding, and Everything In Between* (Facilli, 2023) is an evidence-based approach to all ways of feeding. Written with compassion and a captivating personality, it provides realistic, culturally aware information that empowers families to secure solutions unique to their needs.
2. *Work. Pump. Repeat. The New Mom's Survival Guide to Breastfeeding and Going Back to Work* (Shortall, 2015) prepares parents by sharing relatable stories, including advice on conquering pumping challenges and navigating conversations with human resources before parental leave.
3. *Breastfeeding Made Simple: Seven Natural Laws for Nursing Mothers* (Mohrbacher, Kendall-Tackett, 2010) builds confidence by thoroughly informing parents about what to expect, helping them understand common issues and challenges, and resolving doubts and insecurities.
4. *Readers describe The Womanly Art of Breastfeeding* (Wiessinger, West, Pittman, 2010) as an informative, practical guide covering many topics, including latching, engorgement, safe sleep practices, and night nursing.

Providing adequate breastfeeding support to new mothers and birthing parents is crucial for promoting successful breastfeeding and ensuring the health of both the parent and infant. This support should come from multiple sources, including health care providers, lactation consultants, family members, and community organizations.[19] Proper education on breastfeeding techniques, 1-2-3 positioning, and potential challenges should be provided prenatally and continued after birth.[20] Easily accessible lactation consultants can offer personalized guidance, address concerns, and help overcome obstacles. Support groups allow new parents to share experiences, receive encouragement, and learn from one another. Workplaces should have private lactation rooms and flexibility for pumping breaks.[15] By offering comprehensive practical and emotional support, we can empower mothers and birthing people to meet their breastfeeding goals and give their children the best possible start.

Recognizing disparities in breastfeeding rates among Black women and systemic barriers they face, numerous organizations provide culturally relevant resources and support. Groups like Black Mothers' Breastfeeding Association, Mocha Moms, Chocolate Milk Club, and Mahogany Milk Support Group offer online communities, educational materials, and peer support from Black breastfeeding support specialists; including IBCLCs, CLCs, and peer counselors.[21-23] They create safe spaces celebrating and encouraging breastfeeding while addressing unique challenges Black families encounter. Various organizations strive to increase diversity among lactation consultants and counselors, like the Black Breastfeeding Caucus. An additional key resource consists of an IBCLC sharing one's ethnic background allows culturally competent care, making mothers feel safer, understood, and empowered. Having a circle to openly share triumphs, concerns, and get advice from those understanding the unique cultural context creates powerful solidarity—a reminder mothers are not alone through challenges. By centering Black voices and experiences, they help drive increased breastfeeding initiation and duration rates.[15,19,24,25]

Breastfeeding demands prioritizing self-care as it can be physically and emotionally draining. Simple acts like staying hydrated, eating nutrient-rich foods, getting restful sleep, and taking breaks nourish the mind and body, restoring energy and well-being. Mothers should feel no guilt about carving out "me time" for hobbies, relaxation, or activities bringing joy.[5] Asking partners, friends, or family for help with household duties alleviates burdens.[22] By tending to their needs, all breastfeeding mothers can optimally care for themselves and infants.

In conclusion, navigating the early stages of pregnancy and parenthood involves numerous considerations, from envisioning birth preferences to planning for feeding choices. Prioritizing self-care and adopting healthy habits before pregnancy lays a foundation for both maternal and infant well-being. However, the decision to breast-feed presents its own set of challenges, including the need for adequate support and education. Accessing evidence-based information, receiving support from health care providers, and engaging with peer networks can significantly enhance breast-feeding success. Recognizing and addressing disparities in lactation support, partic-ularly among underrepresented communities, is crucial for promoting equitable access to breastfeeding resources. Ultimately, prioritizing self-care alongside comprehensive support systems empowers parents to navigate the complexities of breastfeeding and nurture their infants with confidence and resilience.

CLINICS CARE POINTS

Preconception Health
- Prioritizing preconception health through a healthy diet, weight management, and physical activity establishes a strong foundation for maternal and infant health. This proactive approach helps manage pregnancy-related challenges and supports long-term well-being.

Support Systems
- Strong support systems from healthcare providers, family, and social networks are essential for breastfeeding success. Comprehensive support enhances maternal self-efficacy and increases the likelihood of achieving breastfeeding goals.

Breastfeeding and Medication
- Lack of clear information or inadequate communication about medication safety can lead to unnecessary discontinuation of breastfeeding or medications. This could negatively impact both the parent's and the infant's health.

Cultural Sensitivity
- Absence of culturally relevant support can alienate families and reduce the effectiveness of breastfeeding guidance. This lack of culturally sensitive care may prevent some families from achieving their breastfeeding goals.

DISCLOSURE

The authors have no conflicts of interest to declare that are relevant to the content of this article.

REFERENCES

1. Marshall NE, Abrams B, Barbour LA, et al. The importance of nutrition in preg-nancy and lactation: lifelong consequences. Am J Obstet Gynecol 2022; 226(5):607–32. https://doi.org/10.1016/j.ajog.2021.12.035.
2. Hill B, Skouteris H, Teede HJ, et al. Health in Preconception, Pregnancy and Post-partum Global Alliance: International Network Preconception Research Priorities

for the Prevention of Maternal Obesity and Related Pregnancy and Long-Term Complications. JCM 2019;8(12):2119. https://doi.org/10.3390/jcm8122119.

3. Grenier LN, Atkinson SA, Mottola MF, et al. Be Healthy in Pregnancy: Exploring factors that impact pregnant women's nutrition and exercise behaviours. Matern Child Nutr 2021;17(1):e13068. https://doi.org/10.1111/mcn.13068.

4. Henshaw EJ, Mayer M, Balraj S, et al. Couples talk about breastfeeding: Interviews with parents about decision-making, challenges, and the role of fathers and professional support. Health Psychol Open 2021;8(2):205510292110291. https://doi.org/10.1177/20551029211029158.

5. McClatchey AK, Shield A, Cheong LH, et al. Why does the need for medication become a barrier to breastfeeding? A narrative review. Women Birth 2018; 31(5):362–6. https://doi.org/10.1016/j.wombi.2017.12.004.

6. Byrne JJ, Saucedo AM, Spong CY. Evaluation of Drug Labels Following the 2015 Pregnancy and Lactation Labeling Rule. JAMA Netw Open 2020;3(8):e2015094. https://doi.org/10.1001/jamanetworkopen.2020.15094.

7. Burkey BW, Holmes AP. Evaluating Medication Use in Pregnancy and Lactation: What Every Pharmacist Should Know. J Pediatr Pharmacol Therapeut 2013;18(3): 247–58. https://doi.org/10.5863/1551-6776-18.3.247.

8. NIH National Library of Medicine. Drugs and lactation database (LactMed®). Bethesda, MD: National Institute of Child Health and Human Development; 2006.

9. Hale's Medications & Mothers' Milk. Available at: https://www.halesmeds.com/. [Accessed 18 March 2024].

10. Beggs B, Koshy L, Neiterman E. Women's Perceptions and Experiences of Breastfeeding: a scoping review of the literature. BMC Publ Health 2021;21: 2169. PMCID: PMC8626903. PMID: 34836514.

11. Lutfiani A, Armini NKA, Kusumaningrum T. Title of the article. J Comput Theor Nanosci 2020;17(7):3053–7. American Scientific Publishers.

12. Marshall NA, Cook CS. Trust Black Women: Using Photovoice to Amplify the Voices of Black Women to Identify and Address Barriers to Breastfeeding in Southeast Georgia. Journal of Health Promotion and Practice 2022;24(1_suppl). https://doi.org/10.1177/15248399221135102.

13. Davis R, Williams J, Chetwynd E. Increasing Diversity in the Field of Lactation: An Interview With the Directors of Pathway 2 IBCLC Programs at Historically Black Colleges and Universities. J Hum Lactation 2021;37(2):230–5.

14. Williams JM. Creating Equity in Lactation Through Historically Black Colleges and Universities. N C Med J 2023;84(1). https://doi.org/10.18043/001c.67789.

15. DeVane-Johnson S, Giscombe CW, Williams II R, et al. A Qualitative Study of Social, Cultural, and Historical Influences on African American Women's Infant-Feeding Practices. J Perinat Educ 2018;27(2):71–85. PMCID: PMC6388681. PMID: 30863005.

16. Tomori C. Overcoming barriers to breastfeeding. Best Pract Res Clin Obstet Gynaecol 2022;83:60–71.

17. Haase B, Brennan E, Wagner CL. Effectiveness of the IBCLC: Have We Made an Impact on the Care of Breastfeeding Families Over the Past Decade? J Hum Lact 2019;35(3):441–52. https://doi.org/10.1177/0890334419851805.

18. Gleason S, Wilkin MK, Sallack L, et al. Breastfeeding Duration Is Associated With WIC Site-Level Breastfeeding Support Practices. J Nutr Educ Behav 2020;52(7): 680–7. https://doi.org/10.1016/j.jneb.2020.01.014.

19. Theodorah DZ, Mc'Deline RN. "The kind of support that matters to exclusive breastfeeding" a qualitative study. BMC Pregnancy Childbirth 2021;21(1):119. https://doi.org/10.1186/s12884-021-03590-2.

20. Piro SS, Ahmed HM. Impacts of antenatal nursing interventions on mothers' breastfeeding self-efficacy: an experimental study. BMC Pregnancy Childbirth 2020;20(1):19. https://doi.org/10.1186/s12884-019-2701-0.

21. Brown A, Shenker N. Experiences of breastfeeding during COVID-19: Lessons for future practical and emotional support. Matern Child Nutr 2021;17(1): e13088. https://doi.org/10.1111/mcn.13088.

22. Emmott EH, Page AE, Myers S. Typologies of postnatal support and breastfeeding at two months in the UK. Soc Sci Med 2020;246:112791. https://doi.org/10.1016/j.socscimed.2020.112791.

23. Gao H, Wang J, An J, et al. Effects of prenatal professional breastfeeding education for the family. Sci Rep 2022;12(1):5577. https://doi.org/10.1038/s41598-022-09586-y.

24. Kehinde J, O'Donnell C, Grealish A. The effectiveness of prenatal breastfeeding education on breastfeeding uptake postpartum: A systematic review. Midwifery 2023;118:103579. https://doi.org/10.1016/j.midw.2022.103579.

25. Parry KC, Tully KP, Hopper LN, et al. Evaluation of Ready, Set, BABY: A prenatal breastfeeding education and counseling approach. Birth 2019;46(1):113–20. https://doi.org/10.1111/birt.12393.

The *Building Respectful Integrated Doula* Support as a *Gateway* for Enhanced Maternal Health Outcomes and *Experiences* Conceptual Framework for Integrating Doula Support in the Pregnancy Continuum

Mulubrhan F. Mogos, PhD, MSc, FAHA[a],*, Rolanda L. Lister, MD[b],
Etoi Garrison, MD[b], Stephanie Devane-Johnson, PhD, CNM[a],
Kristin Mejia, BA, CLC[c], Taneisha Gillyard, PhD[d]

KEYWORDS

- Doula • Pregnancy • Postpartum • Conceptual framework
- Maternal health outcomes

KEY POINTS

- Proven Benefits: Consistent evidence in the literature supports the positive impact of sustained doula support on pregnancy and postpartum outcomes.
- Scalable Model: The *Building Respectful Integrated Doula* Support as a *Gateway* for Enhanced Maternal Health Outcomes and *Experiences* (BRIDGE) framework offers a scalable model for equitable, compassionate, and holistic maternal care, accessible to women across all socioeconomic and ethnic backgrounds.
- Future Research: The BRIDGE framework is expected to guide future research on the benefits of integrating doula support programs in enhancing maternal health outcomes.

INTRODUCTION

The maternal mortality rate in the United States increased by 40% in 2021, making the United States one of the most dangerous places for pregnant women, especially for

[a] Center for Research Development and Scholarship, Vanderbilt University, School of Nursing, Nashville, TN, USA; [b] Department of Obstetrics and Gynecology, Vanderbilt University Medical Center, Nashville, TN, USA; [c] Homeland Heart Birth and Wellness Collective, Nashville, TN, USA; [d] Department of Biomedical Sciences, Meharry Medical College, Nashville, TN, USA
* Corresponding author. Vanderbilt University, School of Nursing, Family Care Community, 21st South Avenue, Nashville, TN 37240.
E-mail address: Mulubrhan.mogos@vanderbilt.edu

Nurs Clin N Am 59 (2024) 527–537
https://doi.org/10.1016/j.cnur.2024.07.001
0029-6465/24/© 2024 Elsevier Inc. All rights reserved, including those for text and data mining, AI training, and similar technologies.

Black and Hispanic pregnant women.[1-3] Doula support has been identified as a cost-saving and effective intervention to improve maternal health.[4-6] Growing number of states are using Medicaid money to integrate doula support as part of the standard of care to improve maternal health outcomes.[7]

Doulas are non-clinical, trained birthing companions who provide emotional, informational, and physical support to pregnant women during the pregnancy continuum (preconception, pregnancy, childbirth, and postpartum periods). This definition does not capture the scope of practice by community-based doulas who are also engaged in providing culturally appropriate support and often are involved in reproductive justice-seeking activism.

Recently, the American College of Obstetricians and Gynecologists and the Society for Maternal-Fetal Medicine acknowledged that sustained doula support during pregnancy improves labor and delivery outcomes.[8-10] However, there is no comprehensive conceptual framework that incorporates the role of doula support across the pregnancy continuum (preconception to postpartum). Therefore, the goal of this article is to review definitions, roles, and outcomes of doula support as well as theoretic/conceptual frameworks used in the context of doula support during the pregnancy continuum, and then use this information to develop a new comprehensive conceptual framework. The newly developed *Building Respectful Integrated Doula Support as a Gateway for Enhanced Maternal Health Outcomes and Experiences (BRIDGE)* framework integrates doula support in the pregnancy continuum and explains the role of doulas as a bridge between providers and patients. The *BRIDGE* framework also details how doulas may complement existing family/social support that, together, may ultimately improve maternal health outcomes and experiences.

THE IMPETUS FOR THE *BUILDING RESPECTFUL INTEGRATED DOULA SUPPORT AS A GATEWAY FOR ENHANCED MATERNAL HEALTH OUTCOMES AND EXPERIENCES* CONCEPTUAL FRAMEWORK
Maternal Morbidity and Mortality Rates in the United States Are Among the Highest in High-Resource Countries

The maternal mortality rate in the United States increased from 23.8 deaths in 2020 to 32.9 deaths per 100,000 live births.[11] For every maternal death, 50 to 100 individuals experience a severe maternal morbidity[12] and continue to live with complex needs including multimorbidity and social deprivation. While the integration of non-clinical interventions such as doula support into usual maternal care has shown promising results in maternal outcomes, including lower rate of cesarean section, short labor duration, less oxytocin use, and positive birth experience,[8-10] there is no comprehensive framework to guide research and practice.

The role of doula support in the pregnancy continuum holds significant promise for improving maternal health outcomes and enhancing overall birthing experiences. This new conceptual framework highlights the diverse roles that doulas can play throughout the entire perinatal journey, complementing existing efforts aimed at enhancing maternal health from pre-conception through postpartum. This framework is also expected to inform future research investigating the impact of implementing doula support integration programs in improving maternal health outcomes. A critical limitation in existing research lies in its focus on the intrapartum period, particularly on reducing cesarean section rate. This lack of comprehensive investigation into the full scope of doula support is partly due to the absence of a framework that outlines the multi-faceted contributions doulas can make across the pregnancy continuum. This proposed framework aims to bridge this gap and serves as a guiding tool for future research developing doula support programs and exploring their impact on birthing experiences and maternal health outcomes.

Maternal Needs During the Pregnancy Continuum Are Not Limited to Clinical Issues

Women of color experience poor maternal health outcomes and are vulnerable to traumatic experiences, a high rate of medical interventions, morbidity, and mortality during pregnancy, childbirth, and postpartum periods. Integrating doulas who are trusted by the community has the potential to provide a crucial support to help pregnant and postpartum women to navigate the complex health care system and receive respectful care.[13] Equally as important is doulas having a deep understanding of the social determinants of health that affect the mothers they serve. These determinants encompass a wide range of interconnected factors such as socioeconomic status, transportation, built environment, housing, and access to quality health care. By actively engaging with mothers and their families along the pregnancy continuum, doulas can address broader contextual factors that influence perinatal health outcomes and connect these families with local resources, empowering mothers to overcome potential barriers to care. For instance, doulas may assist pre-conception or women in early pregnancy in identifying providers who offer culturally appropriate, respectful care, as well as helping to navigate local Medicaid processes in an effort to alleviate some of the financial burden related to maternal health care. They may also connect mothers and their families to nutrition programs or housing assistance. Additionally, doulas with knowledge about neonatal needs can play a pivotal role in guiding new mothers through the early stages of parenthood, fostering critical bonding between mother and child while ensuring a smooth transition through the postpartum period. Doulas, in collaboration with health care providers, can encourage the expansion of support networks beyond the confines of health care facilities by linking mothers to community resources, support groups, and other social services that provide emotional and practical assistance during the perinatal period. Such community connections have been shown to enhance overall maternal well-being, particularly for marginalized populations.[14]

Recently, the coronavirus disease 2019 (COVID-19) pandemic brought about significant changes in maternal care practices, with doulas often perceived as "visitors" and facing restricted access to birthing facilities. However, recent research highlights the indispensable role of doulas in providing essential emotional and informational support, even more so during the challenging times of the COVID-19 pandemic.[15] Moreover, studies have emphasized the importance of community and familial support, particularly for Black mothers whose maternal health outcomes have historically been disproportionately affected by systemic inequities. By acknowledging the invaluable role of doulas in creating a supportive and nurturing environment, health care providers can strengthen the perinatal care experience and potentially improve outcomes, particularly for marginalized populations.

Previously Used Conceptual and Theoretic Frameworks

The integration of doulas into the maternal health care team represents a pivotal advancement in enhancing health outcomes and birth experiences. Previous research underscores the value of continuous emotional and informational support provided by doulas, demonstrating a reduction in interventions and improved overall birth satisfaction.[4] However, the existing literature predominantly focuses on the intrapartum periods, leaving a notable gap in understanding the comprehensive role of doulas across the pregnancy continuum. Similar research highlights the influence of social determinants of health on maternal well-being and how doulas can potentially aid in the disruption of these harmful pathways by providing tailored support and connecting mothers with resources.[13,16,17] Kozhimannil and colleagues utilized the Good Birth Framework which highlights 5 themes that detail how doulas impact pregnancy: agency, personal security, connectedness, respect, and knowledge.[18] While this draws attention to the importance of addressing the broader context within which maternal health unfolds, the specific mechanisms by which doulas integrate into the maternal health care team during the various stages of the pregnancy journey remains widely unexplored.

The BRIDGE framework proposed here seeks to bridge these gaps by presenting a comprehensive approach to doula integration. By positioning doulas as the bridge between health care providers and patients, the framework acknowledges the unique capacity of doulas to provide emotional support, facilitate effective communication and access to respectful care, and empower expectant mothers. As detailed in the conceptual framework presented by Evidence- Based Birth,[19] doulas can play a pivotal role in the intrapartum period, leading to reduced medical interventions and improved birth experiences.[20] However, the BRIDGE framework expands this role to encompass the entire pregnancy continuum, recognizing that support throughout each stage is integral to optimal maternal health outcomes.

Drawing insights from previous research and proposed intrapartum frameworks, the authors present this new conceptual framework for the holistic integration of doulas into the maternal health care team. By encompassing the entire pregnancy continuum and acknowledging and addressing the influence of the many upstream determinants of health, this framework aims to provide a roadmap for health care systems to effectively incorporate doula support in an effort to improve maternal health outcomes and birth experiences.

KEY CONCEPTS IN THE BUILDING RESPECTFUL INTEGRATED DOULA SUPPORT AS A GATEWAY FOR ENHANCED MATERNAL HEALTH OUTCOMES AND EXPERIENCES CONCEPTUAL FRAMEWORK

The BRIDGE framework (**Fig. 1**) is designed to enhance maternal care outcomes by integrating doulas as essential liaisons between health care providers and patients throughout the pregnancy continuum (preconception to 1 year postpartum). Doulas actively engage during preconception, antepartum, intrapartum, and postpartum periods to identify and address barriers that may hinder access to quality care. These barriers encompass various social determinants of health, the built environment, health literacy, and experiences of racism, among others. By recognizing and understanding these barriers, doulas can better advocate for patients and ensure they receive the support they need to access care and resources. Once barriers are identified, doulas play a proactive role in addressing them. This includes assisting patients in overcoming transportation challenges, mobilizing community support networks, providing language assistance, and guiding patients through the complexities of the health care system. By acting as care system navigators, doulas empower patients to navigate the health care landscape effectively, leading to increased patient engagement and better adherence to care plans.

Empowering patient-provider discourse is another key component of the framework. Doulas encourage patients to actively participate in their care decisions, promoting adherence to best practices, self-care recommendations, and regular follow-up visits. This patient-centered approach fosters autonomy and ensures that patients feel respected and involved in their health care choices. Furthermore, doulas play a crucial role in screening for risk factors that may impact maternal health outcomes. They can

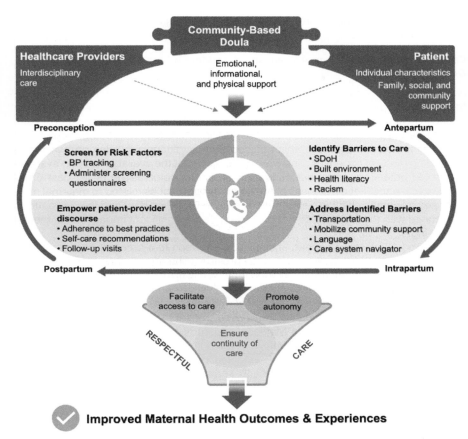

Fig. 1. *B*uilding *R*espectful *I*ntegrated *D*oula *G*ateway for Improved Maternal Health Outcomes and *E*xperience: The *BRIDGE* framework.

measure blood pressure, administer screening questionnaires to assess mental health, and identify potential signs of complications during pregnancy and childbirth. By providing continuous support from preconception to the postpartum period, doulas ensure continuity of care, fostering stronger patient-provider relationships and ultimately leading to improved maternal health outcomes and experiences.

The *BRIDGE* framework emphasizes the critical role doulas play in improving maternal care. By acting as liaisons, addressing barriers, empowering patients, and screening for risk factors, doulas facilitate access to care, promote patient autonomy, and ensure continuity of care throughout the maternal journey. This comprehensive approach to maternal health seeks to enhance outcomes, reduce inequities, and provide respectful, patient-centered care for pregnant and postpartum women.

EXPLAINING THE *B*UILDING *R*ESPECTFUL *I*NTEGRATED *D*OULA SUPPORT AS A *G*ATEWAY FOR ENHANCED MATERNAL HEALTH OUTCOMES AND *E*XPERIENCES FRAMEWORK USING REAL-LIFE EXAMPLES

To illustrate the application of the *BRIDGE* conceptual framework and the impact community doulas may have on birth outcomes and experiences of mothers, the authors describe 2 examples based on qualitative accounts from real mothers who interacted with community doulas.

Case 1: Bridging Gaps for an African American Mom with a Community-Based Doula

A 24-year-old African American woman, residing in a socioeconomically disadvantaged neighborhood, was pregnant for the second time. Her previous pregnancy ended in miscarriage, which left her feeling anxious about navigating the complexities of maternal care once again. She faced the additional challenges of being unemployed and lacking health insurance, which placed a heavy financial burden on her due to impending medical expenses. She was also unaware of the available support systems that could potentially assist her during this time. The combination of her past pregnancy experience, her awareness of the concerning statistics related to maternal mortality and traumatic childbirth experiences among Black women, and the discomforts associated with the first trimester of pregnancy had a significant impact on her mental well-being.

At around 12 weeks pregnant, she still had not been to a prenatal appointment or established a relationship with a perinatal provider. She attended a community baby shower event where she was introduced to a group of Black women who were community-based doulas, whose mission was to serve women just like her in an effort to mitigate the alarming Black maternal mortality rates. She was immediately assigned a caring and dedicated doula who connected her with local resources such as applying for the state's Medicaid program; Women, Infants, and Children Nutrition Program; and Supplemental Nutrition Assistance Program, effectively addressing her financial concerns. The doula performed a comprehensive intake assessment to determine her overall health, knowledge of prenatal care, and potential risk factors. Given the familial and cultural history along with other social determinants of health, it was discussed that there was a likelihood of being at risk for gestational diabetes and hypertension and that once she connected with a provider, the team would work with her to identify preventive measures and/or ensure best practices were followed. Her doula pointed her in the direction of trusted providers and even accompanied her to several prenatal appointments, fostering a sense of empowerment in her medical interactions.

The bond that swiftly formed between the young mother and her doula became the foundation for a transformational partnership rooted in shared experience, cultural understanding, and mutual respect. Along with her partner, they prepared not only for childbirth but also for the complexities of postpartum life. They formulated a birth plan, discussed the mental and emotional challenges that might arise after childbirth, and identified resources that could support her during the postpartum period. The doula emphasized the importance of self-care, taught relaxation techniques, and ensured that the mother felt equipped to recognize any warning signs of postpartum complications, both physical and emotional.

Without the proactive intervention and person-centered guidance provided by her doula, this mother may have continued to traverse the labyrinth of maternal health care alone. The lack of financial resources, appropriate health care access, and fear stemming from her previous miscarriage could have further exacerbated her anxiety, potentially leading to delayed or inadequate prenatal care. This delay might have allowed gestational diabetes or hypertension to go unidentified or unmanaged, posing significant risks to both her and her unborn child. Moreover, without a doula to bridge the communication gap between her and the health care providers, the prenatal visits could have remained intimidating experiences, devoid of the empowerment and advocacy that were critical to her positive maternal experience. The absence of such tailored support and education could have also left her unprepared for the challenges of childbirth and the postpartum period, thus perpetuating a cycle of fear, anxiety, and inadequate care that too many women in socioeconomically disadvantaged situations face.

Case 2: An Immigrant Mom Overcoming Barriers with a Community-Based Doula

Insights gleaned from community-based doulas shed light on the challenges faced by immigrant women in the United States, who frequently encounter not only systemic barriers but also language barriers throughout their pregnancy journeys. In this specific case, the expectant mother was not a native English speaker and resided in a medically underserved area with her older child and an unsupportive partner. While both she and her partner were excited about the impending arrival of their son, she approached the health care system feeling isolated and lacking adequate support. She had been receiving care from an obstetrician but was increasingly frustrated by the communication gaps that hindered effective dialogue. Consequently, she felt that she was struggling to navigate her prenatal care effectively. Her newfound doula, however, shared a similar cultural background and played a crucial role in bridging the language barrier, welcoming her into a supportive community of fellow mothers who could relate to her experiences. The doula also assisted her in deciphering complex medical terminology, bolstering her confidence to actively engage in discussions with her health care providers, and ensuring that her concerns and preferences were clearly conveyed and addressed. Having her doula by her side during labor and delivery ensured seamless communication and left her feeling empowered rather than anxious or fearful.

Following childbirth, she was assigned another doula for the postpartum period. She shared with her doula that she was experiencing intense migraines that seemed to blur her vision. The doula recommended that she check her blood pressure and when they found that it was elevated, the doula suggested that she visit a medical provider as soon as possible. As is common with many mothers, the physiologic changes continued and she was diagnosed with postpartum preeclampsia, a condition not always immediately recognized. Thanks to the doula's training and keen observational skills, the early symptoms including swollen extremities and face, persistent headache, and change in vision were identified. With the doula's guidance, she quickly sought medical care where her health was stabilized, illustrating the invaluable role of the doula beyond the delivery room. After some time, the doula also recognized the signs of mental health struggles and uncovered that the mother was experiencing domestic violence. The doula connected her with organizations specializing in offering support and sanctuary to women in similar situations. Through counseling services and other modes of support, she found both refuge and resilience, highlighting the impact that community-based doulas and their connection to pertinent resources can have on mothers' experiences throughout the pregnancy continuum. The doula also utilized the postpartum meeting as an opportunity to emphasize the significance of preconception care resources available within the community, especially if the patient intends to embark on another pregnancy in the future.

Both of these cases highlight the essential role of community-based doulas in not only addressing systemic gaps but also in tailoring the maternal health care approach to the specific needs of each mother, ultimately facilitating a nurturing, well-informed, and empowered transition into motherhood. Through the *BRIDGE* framework, there lies opportunity to replicate and scale this model, carving a pathway toward equitable,

Table 1
Summary of doula roles during the pregnancy continuum and anticipated outcomes

Timing (Pregnancy Continuum)	Intervention Category	Examples of Recommended Doula Support	Expected Outcomes[a]
Antenatal support	Identify barriers to care and address identified barriers	• Provide information about evidence-based resources • Help completing insurance application if needed • Help patient identify local providers and prepare them with questions to ask their providers. If needed, accompany patient to antenatal care visits	Facilitate access to care; ensure continuity of care
	Empower patient and patient-provider discourse	• Practice breathing techniques, labor positions, and answer questions about the labor process to reduce anxiety	Promote autonomy
	Screen for risk factors	• Assist patients in completing orders prescribed by provider • Administer screening tools (eg, depression scale) and help with home-based blood pressure monitoring	Facilitate access to care; ensure continuity of care
Intrapartum support	Empower patient and patient-provider discourse	• Education about stages of labor • Help with breathing techniques, comfort measures including gentle massage, continuous emotional support to the patient and partner and/or family members • Facilitate communication between patients and their providers.	Promote autonomy
			Ensure continuity of care
Postpartum support	Empower patient and patient-provider discourse	• Help with initiation of breast feeding or bottle feeding, depending on patient preference • Help with scheduling postpartum appointments • Educate about postpartum recovery, interpregnancy interval, infant sleep position, evidence-based resource for preconception care	Promote autonomy; ensure continuity of care
	Empower patient	• Provide support with taking care of older siblings	Facilitate access to care; ensure continuity of care
	Screen for risk factors	• Screen for danger signs including high blood pressure and symptoms of depression	Facilitate access to care; ensure continuity of care

[a] The outcomes are expected to lead to improved pregnancy and postpartum outcomes and experiences.

compassionate, and holistic maternal care for all women, regardless of their socioeconomic or ethnic backgrounds.

DOULA ROLES AND THEIR ASSOCIATION WITH ANTICIPATED OUTCOMES IN ACCORDANCE WITH THE *BUILDING RESPECTFUL INTEGRATED DOULA* SUPPORT AS A *GATEWAY* FOR ENHANCED MATERNAL HEALTH OUTCOMES AND *EXPERIENCES* FRAMEWORK

Within the context of the BRIDGE framework, **Table 1** presents various roles that doulas can undertake to enhance maternal health outcomes and overall childbirth experiences. It is important to note that these illustrative examples are not exhaustive and specific activities performed by doulas can differ, based on their unique training, experience, and polices and guidelines governing doula practice in different localities.

IMPLICATION OF THE *BUILDING RESPECTFUL INTEGRATED DOULA* SUPPORT AS A *GATEWAY* FOR ENHANCED MATERNAL HEALTH OUTCOMES AND *EXPERIENCES* FRAMEWORK IN PRACTICE AND RESEARCH

To effectively integrate doula support into the pregnancy continuum, addressing the educational needs of doulas is paramount. In addition to their crucial role in providing emotional, physical, and informational support to mothers and families throughout the perinatal period, doulas can further ensure their effectiveness through comprehensive and enhanced training.[21] Doulas can aid mothers from low-income and marginalized backgrounds in navigating Medicaid processes. They should also be well-versed in recognizing and responding to the post-birth warning signs as outlined by the Association of Women's Health, Obstetric, and Neonatal Nurses, enabling them to promptly identify potential complications, thereby ensuring timely and appropriate care or referrals.[22]

The literature attests to the positive influence of doulas. However, there is a pressing need for further qualitative and quantitative studies on how doulas directly impact birth outcomes and experiences. Such studies should not only provide narratives on birthing experiences but also data showing the benefits of doula support in improving specific pregnancy outcomes including reduction of unnecessary obstetric procedures, reduction in postpartum depression, reduced length of hospital stay, improved breastfeeding initiation, and the overall maternal experience, among others. The authors believe that the *BRIDGE* conceptual framework can serve as a guide to researchers to determine the timing of doula intervention as well as the timing and type of outcomes to be considered. As we strive to improve maternal outcomes and reduce maternal mortality, nurturing the next generation of doulas through mentorship and guidance by experienced doulas and health care providers is crucial. Researchers and providers should engage with doulas, including community doulas, to identify a common ground where all parties can contribute their fair share toward a healthy pregnancy and pregnancy outcomes.

CLINICS CARE POINTS

- Educational Integration: Prioritize the educational needs of doulas to ensure they are well-prepared to support pregnant and postpartum women effectively throughout the pregnancy continuum.
- Collaborative Engagement: Foster collaboration between researchers, health care providers, and community doulas to establish a shared approach that enhances pregnancy outcomes and promotes a healthy pregnancy.

• Community Trust: Incorporate community-trusted doulas to mitigate mistrust in the health care system, offering essential support that helps women navigate complex health care processes and receive respectful, quality care.

ACKNOWLEDGMENTS

The authors thank Keith Wood, Director of Creative Services and Innovation at Vanderbilt University, School of Nursing for his contribution in designing the conceptual framework.

DISCLOSURE

All authors report no conflict of interest.

FUNDING

This work is partly supported by funding from the Justice-Moore Family Dean's Faculty Fellow Program.

REFERENCES

1. Harris E. US Maternal Mortality Continues to Worsen. JAMA 2023;329(15):1248.
2. Fleszar LG, Bryant AS, Johnson CO, et al. Trends in State-Level Maternal Mortality by Racial and Ethnic Group in the United States. JAMA 2023;330(1):52–61.
3. Abbasi J. US Maternal Mortality Is Unacceptably High, Unequal, and Getting Worse—What Can Be Done About It? JAMA 2023;330(4):302–5.
4. Dekker R. Evidence on: Doulas. Available at: https://evidencebasedbirth.com/the-evidence-for-doulas/. [Accessed 13 September 2023].
5. Kozhimannil KB, Hardeman RR, Alarid-Escudero F, et al. Modeling the cost-effectiveness of doula care associated with reductions in preterm birth and cesarean delivery. Birth 2016;43(1):20–7.
6. Falconi AM, Bromfield SG, Tang T, et al. Doula care across the maternity care continuum and impact on maternal health: Evaluation of doula programs across three states using propensity score matching. EClinicalMedicine 2022;50:101531.
7. Chen A. Current State of Doula Medicaid Implementation Efforts in November 2022. 2023. Available at: https://healthlaw.org/current-state-of-doula-medicaid-implementation-efforts-in-november-2022/.
8. ACOG Committee Opinion No. 766 Summary: approaches to limit intervention during labor and birth. Obstet Gynecol 2019;133(2):406–8.
9. Bohren MA, Hofmeyr GJ, Sakala C, et al. Continuous support for women during childbirth. Cochrane Database Syst Rev 2017;(7). https://doi.org/10.1002/14651858. CD003766.pub6.
10. Kennell J, Klaus M, McGrath S, et al. Continuous emotional support during labor in a US hospital. A randomized controlled trial. JAMA 1991;265(17):2197–201.
11. DL H. Maternal mortality rates in the United States, 2021. NCHS Health E-Stats. 2021. doi: https://dx.doi.org/10.15620/cdc:124678 October 19, 2023. Available at: https://www.cdc.gov/nchs/data/hestat/maternal-mortality/2021/maternal-mortality-rates-2021.htm#:~:text=The%20maternal%20mortality%20rate%20for,20.1%20in%202019%20(Table).
12. Geller SE, Koch AR, Garland CE, et al. A global view of severe maternal morbidity: moving beyond maternal mortality. Reprod Health 2018/06/22 2018;15(1):98.

13. Kozhimannil KB, Vogelsang CA, Hardeman RR, et al. Disrupting the pathways of social determinants of health: doula support during pregnancy and childbirth. J Am Board Fam Med 2016;29(3):308–17.
14. Balaji AB, Claussen AH, Smith DC, et al. Social support networks and maternal mental health and well-being. J Womens Health (Larchmt) 2007;16(10):1386–96.
15. Adams C. Pregnancy and birth in the United States during the COVID-19 pandemic: The views of doulas. Birth 2022;49(1):116–22.
16. Mottl-Santiago J, Dukhovny D, Cabral H, et al. Effectiveness of an enhanced community doula intervention in a safety net setting: a randomized controlled trial. Health Equity 2023;7(1):466–76.
17. Marudo C, Nicotra C, Fletcher M, et al. Bridging health disparities and improving reproductive outcomes with health center-affiliated doula programs. Obstet Gynecol 2023;142(4):886–92.
18. Springen K. A good birth: finding the positive and profound in your childbirth experience. Booklist 2013;109(22):15.
19. Dekker R. Evidence-based birth: Putting current evidence based information into the hands of communities, so they can make empowered choices. Available at: https://evidencebasedbirth.com/. [Accessed 12 October 2023].
20. Landor C. Right to informed consent, right to a doula: an evidence-based solution to the black maternal mortality crisis in the United States. Mich J Gend Law 2023;30:61.
21. Broussard, Libertie and Mejia-Greene, Kristen and Devane-Johnson, Stephanie and Lister, Rolanda, Collaborative Training as a Conduit to Build Knowledge in Black Birth Workers. Available at: https://ssrn.com/abstract=4126902 or https://doi.org/10.2139/ssrn.4126902.
22. Suplee PD, Kleppel L, Santa-Donato A, Bingham D. Improving postpartum education about warning signs of maternal morbidity and mortality. Nurs Womens Health 2017;20:552–67.

Comprehensive Care in the Fourth Trimester
A Guide for Nurses

Jacquelyn McMillian-Bohler, PhD, CNM, CNE[a],*,
Bonnie Jones-Hepler, PhD, MSW, MSPH, RN[b],
Melissa Katella, MSN, RN, CNE[c],
Stephanie Gedzyk-Nieman, DNP, RNC-MNN[b]

KEYWORDS

- Fourth trimester • BUBBLE-LE framework • Postpartum • Breastfeeding
- Post partum assessment • Newborn assessment • Sexual health

KEY POINTS

- The period from birth to 12 weeks postpartum, known as the fourth trimester, includes significant events such as physical, hormonal, and emotional changes for birthing persons and developmental milestones for infants.
- Nurses play a crucial role in supporting both physical and emotional recovery during the fourth trimester.
- Regular screenings and support for postpartum emotional health, including postpartum depression and anxiety, is essential for overall well-being.
- Effective breastfeeding support and guidance regarding infant care are vital. Specific guidance may include education on proper techniques, comfort measures, and recognizing developmental milestones to support both feeding and sleeping routines.
- Engaging the birthing person's partner and family in postpartum care plans and utilizing resources such as postpartum doulas and educational programs like the Fourth Trimester Project enhance support for new families, improving overall outcomes during this transitional period.

While childbirth is typically divided into 3 antepartum trimesters, a modern understanding of childbearing care acknowledges the significance of the fourth trimester, extending from birth to 12 weeks postpartum. During this period, new mothers undergo significant physical changes, including uterine involution and the healing of lacerations or surgical incisions, and hormonal adjustments.[1] Additionally, new parents

[a] Department of Nursing, Duke University School of Nursing, 307 Trent Drive, Durham, NC 27710, USA; [b] Duke University School of Nursing, 307 Trent Drive, Durham, NC 27710, USA; [c] Duke University Health System, 307 Trent Drive, Durham, NC 27710, USA
* Corresponding author.
E-mail address: Jmm234@duke.edu

Nurs Clin N Am 59 (2024) 539–550
https://doi.org/10.1016/j.cnur.2024.08.004
nursing.theclinics.com

face challenges including role transitions, sleep disturbances, and the demands of newborn care.

Nurses play a pivotal role in supporting patients throughout the entire birthing process. By offering anticipatory guidance, follow-up care, and advocacy, nurses can significantly enhance the well-being of both new mothers and their infants. This paper describes practical insights and strategies for effective nursing care during the fourth trimester.

CARE IN THE FOURTH TRIMESTER

Support for birthing individuals and their families is just as critical in the weeks following birth as it is during pregnancy.[2] The postpartum period presents unique challenges, including physical recovery, emotional transitions, parenting hurdles, and shifts in family dynamics. Data indicate that 42% of maternal mortality occurs postpartum,[3] however during this period, contact with health care providers is often limited to 1 or 2 scheduled visits. Comprehensive and effective postpartum care is essential to prevent and manage potential complications arising after childbirth[4] thus this lack of interaction is inadequate.

Infants also experience important developmental milestones and establish feeding and sleep patterns during the fourth trimester. Traditionally, childbirth education has focused primarily on antepartum visits, with limited follow-up during the postpartum period. This gap often leaves new parents to manage their needs on their own during a crucial and complex period, resulting in unmet needs and increased stress.

Nurses provide education, discharge teaching, and often follow-up with patients, triaging calls when families have questions. They can be an important link in improving outcomes for postpartum patients. The following sections outline specific assessments and interventions nurses can perform to provide quality care to both the birthing persons and the infant during the fourth trimester.

KEY AREAS OF FOCUS FOR NURSING CARE
General Postpartum Assessments of the Birthing Person

In the immediate postpartum period, close monitoring of vital signs is essential. Blood pressures should align with pre-pregnancy baseline levels. Elevated blood pressure may suggest preeclampsia, while lower levels, particularly with tachycardia, could indicate a significant hemorrhage. A temperature up to 100.4°F is normal in the first 24 hours due to possible dehydration, but higher temperatures, especially with tachycardia, may signal an infection.

Physical Assessments

Traditionally, nurses have used the acronym *BUBBLE-LE* to organize postpartum assessments. The BUBBLE-LE framework provides a valuable structure for conducting a thorough assessment of the postpartum parent. However, it's essential to understand that the assessments do not need to follow the exact sequence outlined in the framework. For instance, during an interaction with a postpartum parent, obtaining consent first and starting with less intrusive assessments, such as checking extremities or asking about voiding, can foster a more respectful and comfortable experience for the parent.

- Breasts: Inspect for infection or nipple trauma and palpate for fullness, pain, or tenderness.

- Uterus: Palpate the fundus to assess involution. It should be firm, midline, and progressively return to baseline. Deviations may suggest a full bladder or increased risk of hemorrhage.
- Bladder: Ensure the patient can void easily and check for signs of urinary tract infection.
- Bowel: Check for active bowel sounds and offer interventions to prevent constipation.
- Lochia: Assess the amount and characteristics of lochia, which should be red (rubra) for 1 to 3 days, pink/brown (serosa) for 3 to 10 days, and yellow/white (alba) thereafter. The amount should decrease daily, remain odorless, and clots should be smaller than an egg. Deviations may indicate infection or hemorrhage.
- Episiotomy/Perineum: Inspect for intactness, bruising, edema, redness, discharge, and hematomas. Also, check for hemorrhoids.
- Lower Extremities: Examine for redness, unilateral edema, and calf pain to detect potential thrombus formation. Implement preventive measures like early ambulation and pneumatic compression devices.
- Emotions: Emotional and psychological assessments will be discussed later in this article.

Pain Management

Common postpartum pains include uterine, perineal, rectal (from hemorrhoids), and incisional (post-cesarean). Postpartum pain is typically managed with a combination of oral and topical medications, such as those for hemorrhoids and perineal discomfort. Non-pharmacological interventions can also be beneficial, including perineal ice packs for the first 24 to 48 hours, sitz baths, and abdominal binders. Patients should be instructed to notify providers if pain is not relieved with prescribed medications or if pain continues to get progressively worse.

Postpartum Health Issues

Up to 10% of birthing persons can experience health issues in the postpartum period, including hypertension, thyroid disorders, and diabetes.[5] Patients who have experienced complications related to these disorders will be monitored during the postpartum period. However, some patients may develop new complications, and therefore, should receive education about the signs and symptoms so that they can follow-up if any complications occur.

Emotional and Psychological Support

Becoming a parent can bring immense joy, but it also involves significant change and intense emotions. The postpartum period includes expected emotional shifts, such as postpartum blues (or "baby blues"). However, conditions like postpartum depression (PPD) and anxiety are less expected and require additional intervention to prevent negative outcomes. Mental health issues are a leading cause of postpartum mortality.[6] While approximately 80% of new parents experience postpartum blues[7] about 12% face postpartum[8,9] Unlike PPD, postpartum blues are short-lived, peaking around the fifth day and resolving by the tenth day. In contrast, PPD can develop at any point within the first year after delivery, typically emerging between 2 and 12 weeks postpartum.

At a minimum, clients should be screened for depression and other mental health conditions immediately postpartum, at 6 weeks, and at 2, 4, and 6-months postbirth[10] Screening at every well-child visit during the first year can also be beneficial. The Edinburgh Postnatal Depression Scale (EPDS) is the most widely used tool. Its advantages include its brevity (10 items), free availability, and coverage of anxiety, depressive symptoms, and suicidal ideation. A total score of 9 or higher, or a score of 1 or greater on the item related to suicidal thoughts, indicates the need for referral to a mental health professional for diagnosis and treatment[9] Since 2021, the rates of death by suicide have increased in the postpartum period. Up to 20% of maternal deaths in the postpartum period are attributed to death by suicide.[11]

Nurses play a crucial role in providing emotional support and education, as well as connecting patients with necessary mental health resources. Patients may feel ashamed of their emotions and need reassurance that their feelings are not their fault. Educating them about sleep promotion (for both them and their infants), stress management, and self-care can positively impact their mental health and overall well-being.[10]

The comprehensive care provided by nurses extends beyond emotional support and education; it encompasses all facets of postpartum well-being, including sexual health. As trusted health care professionals, nurses are uniquely positioned to address the often-neglected topic of sexual health, ensuring that it is integrated into the holistic care plan for new mothers.

Sexual Health Assessments in the Postpartum Period

Sexual health is a crucial aspect of postpartum care, but it is often overlooked.[12] Research indicates that approximately 1 in 3 women experiences dyspareunia, or painful intercourse, within the first 6 months postpartum. A meta-analysis by Cattani and colleagues[13] reported that sexual dysfunction may not be exclusive to vaginal births, as patients who gave birth by cesarean section also experienced dysfunction. Additionally, some birthing perscons report a decreased libido, which may be attributed to hormonal changes or exhaustion from caring for a newborn[14] Neglecting sexual health can negatively impact relationships and overall well-being. It is crucial for birthing individuals to be informed about all available options, including their associated risks and benefits, to make well-informed decisions about their sexual and reproductive health. Nurses can use assessment tools such as the *PLISSIT model* to facilitate discussions about sexual health.[15] The *PLISSIT model* includes:

- Permission: Encourage clients to talk openly about sexual health by giving them explicit permission to discuss their concerns.
- Limited Information: Provide relevant information that addresses specific issues or questions the client may have.
- Specific Suggestions: Offer tailored advice to improve problems or challenges related to sexual health.
- Intensive Therapy: Refer clients to specialized therapy, including pelvic physical therapy if needed, for more in-depth support and treatment.

While discussions on family planning and sexual health are essential, the postpartum period also demands attention to breastfeeding. Nurses play a pivotal role in educating and supporting new parents, ensuring both the well-being of the birthing individual and the nutritional needs of the infant are met.

Breastfeeding Support

For birthing clients who choose to breast or chest-feed their newborns, education and encouragement are crucial. In the initial days post-birth, when a mature milk supply has not yet been established, proper technique and support are key to increasing the likelihood of successful, long-term breastfeeding. The American Academy of Pediatrics[16] recommends exclusive breastfeeding (whether at the breast/chest or expressed) for the first 6 months of life. However, around 60% of breastfeeding clients do not meet their intended breastfeeding duration. Common reasons for discontinuation include difficulties with latching, cultural practices, insufficient family or community support, concerns about the infant's well-being (often related to perceived insufficient milk supply), and the challenges of returning to work without adequate support for milk expression.[17]

To support breastfeeding clients effectively, it is recommended to feed their newborns on demand rather than adhering to a strict schedule. Health care providers should encourage feeding 8 to 12 times in a 24-hr period, based on the newborn's hunger cues. Parents should be advised to recognize signs such as an awake and alert state, mouth movements like opening and closing, lip-smacking, tongue ejection, an engaged rooting reflex, bringing hands to the mouth, and crying (a late sign of hunger) as indicators that it's time to feed. Frequent skin-to-skin contact and allowing the newborn to stay with the feeding parent post-birth can also enhance breastfeeding success, aligning with national recommendations.[18]

Support from both professionals (such as nurses and lactation consultants) and lay personnel is essential for breastfeeding success.[19] Addressing issues like painful latching, cluster feeding, and assessing if the newborn is getting enough milk is particularly important in the early days. Ensuring a deep latch, where the newborn takes the areola into their mouth with their mouth wide open and lips flanged, can alleviate nipple pain associated with shallow latching. Proper latching, combined with comfort measures for the feeding parent and adequate breast/chest support during feeding, helps prevent nipple discomfort and damage.[19,20]

Comfort Measures for Breastfeeding

To alleviate sore nipples, several comfort measures can be effective.[20]

- Topical Treatments: Lanolin creams, non-lanolin alternatives like coconut oil, hydrogel pads, and silver nipple shields can help soothe and protect the nipples. A mild analgesic, such as ibuprofen, may also provide relief.
- Self-Care: Expressing colostrum or breast milk and applying it to the sore area can promote healing. Allowing the area to air-dry can also be beneficial.

Health care providers should assess the infant's oral cavity, the feeding parent's nipple anatomy, and the overall feeding technique to offer tailored advice and support for a more comfortable feeding experience. Adjusting feeding positions can also alleviate nipple pain.

For clients experiencing engorgement, the following measures can enhance comfort.

- Pre-Feeding: Apply moist heat to the breast or chest for 10 minutes to facilitate milk flow.
- During Feeding: Hand express milk to soften the areolar tissue and gently massage the engorged area.
- Post-Feeding: Apply ice to the breast or chest for 10 to 15 minutes to reduce swelling and discomfort.

Nurses may provide lactation consult and make recommendations for lactation support as needed. Some birthing persons may discontinue breast feeding during the fourth trimester period and may need support during the weaning process. In addition to lactation support for the birthing person, nurses provide newborn assessments that ensure a healthy start for the infant.

INFANT CARE
Newborn Assessments

The initial newborn assessment is conducted within the first few minutes of life to evaluate the need for immediate interventions using the APGAR scoring system. During the immediate postpartum period, frequent assessments ensure the newborn's continued transition to extrauterine life.[21]

Key Assessments Include

- Vital Signs:
  - Heart rate: normal 110 to 160 bpm
  - Respiratory rate: normal 30 to 60 breaths per minute
  - Temperature: normal 36.5 to 37.4°C
  - Blood pressure and oxygen saturation are not routinely assessed unless medically indicated.
  - Pre-ductal and post-ductal oxygenation are checked to complete the critical congenital heart disease (CCHD) screening at 24 hours of life.
- Newborn Measurements:
  - Weight
  - Length
  - Head, chest, and neck circumferences

Routine and recommended newborn medications are typically administered during the first nursing assessment, within the first 1 to 2 hours of life.

- Medications:
  - Vitamin K (phytonadione): Given intramuscularly to prevent vitamin K deficiency bleeding.
  - Erythromycin ophthalmic ointment: Applied to prevent gonococcal conjunctivitis.
  - Hepatitis B vaccine: The first dose is recommended within the first 24 hours to prevent long-term hepatitis B infection.

A complete cephalocaudal assessment should be performed, examining:

- Overall appearance, including skin, head, neck, chest, trunk, abdomen, genitalia, anus, extremities, and spine.
- Neurologic status, including common newborn reflexes (Moro, sucking, rooting, stepping, palmar and plantar grasp, Babinski).

Document any variations in assessment findings, such as a heart murmur, which may be transient and physiologically normal. Considerations during the assessment include:

- Maintaining infant comfort
- Ensuring thermoregulation
- Encouraging family-centered involvement
- Recording infant intake and output as part of ongoing assessments

Newborn Follow-up

In contrast to common maternal postpartum follow-up appointments, newborns typically have very close and frequent follow-up in the fourth trimester. The American Academy[22] of Pediatrics recommends a newborn not be discharged without scheduled follow-up in 24 to 48 hours of discharge. Newborns typically regain their birth weight by 10 to 14 days of life. Route of delivery and type of feeding (human milk vs formula) may impact regaining of birth weight, in relation to the amount of weight lost after the first 3 to 5 days of life.

Infant Feeding

During the early postpartum period, feeding often occupies the thoughts and energy of parents. Current recommendations around feeding include.[23]

- Striving for skin-to-skin contact between the birthing parent and infant immediately postpartum.
- Cue-based feeding for infants fed with human milk.
- Monitoring of infant output, growth, and behaviors to ensure appropriate feeding.

Feeding times offer valuable opportunities for infants and their caregivers to interact. It is ideal to hold an infant during feedings for both developmental and safety reasons. Parents often have concerns about whether their infant is feeding enough, as well as about gas and spit-up. Techniques to help relieve discomfort for the infant include.

- Stomach massage
- Pace bottle feeding
- Bicycling infant legs
- Watching for infant satiation cues

Meeting feeding goals often depends on the extent to which the larger system around the family supports the dyad. Nurses frequently face difficult discussions when recommendations and standards of practice are not aligned with the family's culture, values, or circumstances. Examples include.

- Introduction of pumping before establishing infant feeding
- Use of certain substances while lactating
- Not boiling water prior to reconstituting formula

In such cases, it is the nurse's responsibility to thoughtfully communicate current recommendations and their rationales while allowing for shared decision-making, which could lead to harm reduction conversations as needed.

Sleep Patterns

Establishing good sleep hygiene routines during the early postpartum period is essential for promoting maternal well-being. This is especially challenging for parents who face pressures to return to work and other responsibilities before their child can develop circadian rhythms. Transformative shifts in the expectations of newly postpartum parents, such as the widespread adoption of parental leave, are needed. However, in the interim, numerous nursing actions can assess and support sleep during the postpartum period.

- Maternal perception of sleep appears to be a stronger driver of maternal mental health outcomes than objective measures such as actigraphy. Therefore, nurses should ask questions like "How have you been sleeping?" rather than "How much sleep are you getting?"
- Having a support system that shares nighttime infant care responsibilities and ensures at least one 3 to 4 hour protected, uninterrupted block of sleep is essential for maternal well-being.
- Teaching fathers and other caregivers about infant behavior and ways to meet the infant's needs without intervention from the birthing parent builds family

capacity. Engaging additional caregivers acknowledges their unique strengths in the child's life.

Finally, as with feeding, cultural practices or personal preferences (e.g., bed sharing, infant sleeping in a separate room from parents) may not align with current recommendations for safe sleep practices as outlined by the American Academy of Pediatrics. These are difficult conversations that require a nurse to fully understand the benefits of the recommendations and engage in thoughtful harm reduction conversations when gold standard recommendations are not the preferred practice of the family.[24]

Highlighting Infant Behavior During Nursing Assessments

Institutions like the Brazelton Institute offer comprehensive courses on using physical assessments to help parents understand infant behavior.[25] A nurse's narration of their observations during a physical assessment can be instrumental in helping families decode their infant's behavior.

Infant states such as quiet sleep, active sleep, drowsiness, quiet alert, active alert, and crying are important indicators of the infant's current condition and needs.[25] Assessment findings based on engagement, including ball tracking and hearing responses, can provide insights into the infant's sensory development and interaction with their environment. Reflexes, such as the palmar grasp, play a significant role in the infant's development. For example, the palmar grasp reflex helps the baby hold onto objects, fostering curiosity and exploration of their surroundings.

When conducting an infant assessment, if an infant is in a quiet alert state, a nurse could explain that the infant may enjoy tracking a bright ball or exploring a noisy rattle. As this is demonstrated, the nurse also gathers assessment data on hearing and vision. Similarly, if a family needs to help an infant transition from a sleeping state to an alert state, a nurse may help the family understand how their infant responds to light or sound (e.g, habituation). Infants constantly communicate and explore the world around them, and as a nurse, it is a privilege to decode those behaviors, highlighting each infant's particular interests and strengths.

Infant Crying

In the modern world, infants can experience significant overstimulation as they become increasingly aware of their surroundings, sometimes leading to periods of PURPLE crying (Peak of Crying, Unexpected, Resists soothing, Pain-like face, Long lasting, Evening). It is essential to support parental well-being during these times.[26] Nurses can advise caregivers to try strategies such as having others hold their infant during crying bouts; or placing the infant in a safe place while the caregiver takes a brief respite if feeling stressed.

Emphasizing the importance of self-care, nurses can reassure caregivers that managing their stress is essential so they can be fully present and attentive to their infant's needs once they resume caregiving.

Toward the end of the 4th trimester, nurses can offer anticipatory guidance, noting that infants may exhibit disorganized behavior right before they learn a new skill (eg, crawling, sitting, walking). Remind parents to rule out sickness and other discomforts (like teething), but also that sleep regressions or behavior changes might indicate a rapid period of learning for the infant.

Caregiver-infant relationships: early relational health

Relationships between caregivers and their infants are dynamic. One significant critique of theories like attachment theory is that labeling a child as securely attached

Table 1
Summary of nursing care in the fourth trimester

Fourth Trimester Assessments	Key Interventions
Postpartum Assessment	• BUBBLE-LE: (B)Breasts, (U)Uterus (fundus), (B)Bladder, (B)Bowel, (L) Lochia, (E)Episiotomy (perineum), (L)Lower leg, and (E)Emotions.
Pain	• Oral medications • Topical medications (for hemorrhoids and perineal discomforts) • Perineal ice packs for the first 24–48 h post-birth • Sitz baths • Abdominal binders
Mental Health	• At minimum, screen clients in the immediate postpartum period, at 6 wk, and 2, 4, and 6-mo post-birth • Reassure the client their feelings are not their fault • Provide education on sleep promotion (self and infant), stress management, and self-care
Sexual Health	Use the PLISSIT model to assess sexual health. (P) Permission; (L) Limited information; (SP) Specific Suggestions; (IP) Intensive Therapy
Support	• Help the family identify all support options • Encourage the inclusion of the partner in postpartum plans • Educate both the birthing person and the partner about newborn care and postpartum recovery • Inform the family about resources like the Fourth Trimester Project • Suggest considering a postpartum doula for additional support

Newborn Assessment	• Vital Signs:
	  ○ Heart rate: normal 110–160 bpm
	  ○ Respiratory rate: normal 30–60 breaths per minute
	  ○ Temperature: normal 36.5–37.4°C
	  ○ Blood pressure and oxygen saturation are not routinely assessed unless medically indicated.
	  ○ Pre-ductal and post-ductal oxygenation are checked to complete the critical congenital heart disease (CCHD) screening at 24 h of life
	• Newborn Measurements:
	  ○ Weight
	  ○ Length
	  ○ Head, chest, and neck circumferences
	  ○ These measurements are recorded for growth monitoring and plotted on the WHO growth curve.

Feeding	• *Skin-to-Skin Contact*: Encourage skin-to-skin contact between the birthing parent and infant immediately after birth. • *Cue-Based Feeding*: Promote cue-based feeding for human milk-fed infants, paying attention to infant output, growth, and behaviors. • *Interaction Opportunities*: Feeding times provide valuable opportunities for infants and caregivers to interact. Holding the infant during feedings is ideal for both developmental and safety reasons. • *Parental Concerns*: Address parents' questions about whether their infant is feeding enough and address concerns about gas and spit-up. • *Discomfort Relief Techniques*: After ruling out allergies or intolerances, demonstrate techniques such as stomach massage, pace bottle feeding, bicycling infant legs, and watching infant satiation cues. • *Challenges and Communication*: Recognize that meeting feeding goals depends on the larger family system's support. Nurses may face

(continued on next page)

Table 1 (continued)	
Fourth Trimester Assessments	**Key Interventions**
	difficult discussions when recommendations clash with cultural values or circumstances. Thoughtful communication and shared decision-making are essential in such cases.
Sleep	• *Assess Sleep Perception*: Instead of just asking about the number of hours of sleep, inquire about how the parent perceives their sleep quality. This can provide valuable insights into their mental well-being.
	• *Promote Support Systems*: Encourage birthing parents to establish a support system for nighttime infant care. Sharing responsibilities ensures that parents get uninterrupted sleep.
	• *Educate Caregivers*: Teach fathers and other caregivers about infant behavior and ways to meet the infant's needs independently. This builds family capacity and acknowledges unique strengths.
	• *Navigate Cultural Practices*: When cultural practices or personal preferences conflict with safe sleep recommendations, engage in thoughtful conversations. Understand the benefits of recommendations and explore harm reduction strategies if needed.

fails to account for the constantly changing relationship between the caregiver and child. Similarly, the concept of bonding emphasizes the outward expression of a dyad's relationship at a moment in time. However, leaders in Early Relational Health now emphasize concepts like "The Good Enough Parent," focusing not on being the perfect parent but on being a responsive, caring parent who addresses infant needs as they arise.[27]

Being responsive to these needs does not spoil an infant. Instead, these moments are crucial for infants, reinforcing the idea that "if I have a need, my caregiver helps me." Striving to be the perfect parent is unnecessary because it deprives the infant of learning who helps them when they have needs and how that person helps. Parents should aim to be caring and responsive, not perfect. This approach helps nurses adopt a non-judgmental, collaborative stance and support parents who may struggle with parental guilt or self-doubt.

Support for the Birthing Person

It is important to include the birthing person's partner in postpartum plans. The partner will assist in caring for the newborn and can be a source of emotional support for the birthing person. The partner may be the person most often with the birthing person and can offer another source for assessment of any complications that may arise. Other members of the family can also provide significant support.[28] Often, education is only provided to the birthing person, missing an opportunity to involve the partner. As a result, the partner may not feel fully included or equipped to support the birthing person effectively.

Programs such as the Fourth Trimester Project,[28] can be used as prompts to assist the family in considering how they would like to be supported during the postpartum period. A postpartum doula is another resource that may be available to some families. A doula can assist with the care of the newborn and provide physical and emotional support for the recovering birthing person. The nurse should help the family to identify all their support options (**Table 1**).

SUMMARY

Comprehensive care during the fourth trimester is crucial for the well-being of both birthing individuals and their infants. This period, which extends from birth to 12 weeks postpartum, involves significant physical, hormonal, and emotional changes that require attentive and holistic nursing care. Nurses play a vital role not only in physical assessments but also in providing emotional support, pain management, and education on infant care. Using the BUBBLE-LE framework helps ensure thorough monitoring of physical recovery and emotional health. Addressing conditions such as postpartum depression, breastfeeding issues, and sexual health concerns is essential for preventing complications and improving the postpartum experience. Involving partners and family members[28] and utilizing resources like postpartum doulas can enhance support. Educational programs, such as the Fourth Trimester Project, offer valuable tools for families navigating this transition. Ultimately, effective postpartum care depends on a collaborative approach involving health care providers, partners, and support networks. Prioritizing comprehensive, empathetic care helps improve outcomes for birthing individuals and their families during this critical period.

DISCLOSURE

The authors have no known disclosures.

REFERENCES

1. Mehta A, Srinivas SK. The fourth trimester: 12 Weeks is not enough. Obstet Gynecol 2021;137(5):779–81.
2. Montgomery TM, Laury E. A call for comprehensive care in the fourth trimester. Nursing for Women's Health 2019;23(3):194–9.
3. Hoyert DL. Maternal mortality rates in the United States, 2021, National Center for Health Statistics (U.S) 2023. https://dx.doi.org/10.15620/cdc:124678.
4. Quebedeaux TM, Holman S. The fourth trimester: embracing the chaos of the postpartum period. TOJ 2024;24(2):93–5.
5. Paladine HL, Blenning CE, Strangas Y. Postpartum care: an approach to the fourth trimester. Am Fam Physician 2019;100(8):485–91.
6. Trost SL, Beauregard J, Njie F, et al. Pregnancy-Related Deaths: Data from Maternal Mortality Review Committees in 36 US States, 2017–2019. Atlanta, GA: Centers for Disease Control and Prevention, US Department of Health and Human Services; 2022.
7. March of Dimes, Baby blues after pregnancy, Available at: https://www.marchofdimes.org/find-support/topics/postpartum/baby-blues-after-pregnancy, (Accessed 11 July 2024), 2021.
8. Bauman BL, Ko JY, Cox S, et al. Vital signs: postpartum depressive symptoms and provider discussions about perinatal depression - United States, 2018. MMWR Morb Mortal Wkly Rep 2020;69(19):575–81.
9. Cox JL, Holden JM, Sagovsky R. Detection of postnatal depression. Development of the 10-item Edinburgh postnatal depression Scale. Br J Psychiatry 1987;150:782–6.
10. Gedzyk-Nieman SA. Postpartum and paternal postnatal depression: identification, risks, and resources. Nurs Clin North Am 2021;56(3):325–43.
11. CDC, Pregnancy-related deaths: data from maternal mortality review committees in 36 U.S. States, 2017–2019. Maternal Mortality Prevention, Available at: https://

www.cdc.gov/maternal-mortality/php/data-research/mmrc-2017-2019.html, (Accessed 11 July 2024), 2024.

12. Graziottin A, Di Simone N, Guarano A. Postpartum care: clinical considerations for improving genital and sexual health. Eur J Obstet Gynecol Reprod Biol 2024;296:250–7.

13. Cattani L, De Maeyer L, Verbakel JY, et al. Predictors for sexual dysfunction in the first year postpartum: a systematic review and meta-analysis. BJOG 2022;129(7): 1017–28.

14. Grussu P, Vicini B, Quatraro RM. Sexuality in the perinatal period: a systematic review of reviews and recommendations for practice. Sex Reprod Healthc 2021;30:100668.

15. Carroll CC, Trotter KJ, McMillian-Bohler J, et al. Improving perinatal sexual health assessment: PLISSIT model implementation. Womens Healthc 2022;10(6):46–9.

16. American Academy of Pedicatrics. Newborn and infant breastfeeding. Available at: https://www.aap.org/en/patient-care/newborn-and-infant-nutrition/newborn-and-infant-breastfeeding/. (Accessed 11 July 2024).

17. U.S. Department of Health & Human Services. Breastfeeding: facts. Centers for Disease Control and Prevention. 2023. Available at: https://www.cdc.gov/breast feeding/data/facts.html#indicators.

18. Bureau UC. Maternity leave and employment patterns of first-time mothers: 1961-2008. Available at: Census.gov. Accessed July 29, 2024 https://www.census.gov/library/publications/2011/demo/p70-128.html.

19. Cohen SS, Alexander DD, Krebs NF, et al. Factors associated with breastfeeding initiation and continuation: a meta-analysis. J Pediatr 2018;203:190–6.e21.

20. Gavine A, Shinwell SC, Buchanan P, et al. Support for healthy breastfeeding mothers with healthy term babies. Cochrane Pregnancy and Childbirth Group. Cochrane Database Syst Rev 2022;2022(10). https://doi.org/10.1002/14651858. CD001141.pub6.

21. Baker B, Janke J. Core curriculum for maternal-newborn nursing. In: McKeee G, editor. UpToDate. 6th edition. Missouri: Elsevier; 2024. Available at: https://www.uptodate.com/contents/assessment-of-the-newborn-infant. Accessed July 29, 2024.

22. Association of Women's Health, Obstetric and Neonatal Nurses (AWHONN). Breastfeeding and the use of human milk. J Obstet Gynecol Neonatal Nurs 2021; 50(5):e1–5.

23. Moon RY, Carlin RF, Hand I, The Task Force on Sudden Infant Death Syndrome and the Committee on Fetus and Newborn. Sleep-related infant deaths: updated 2022 recommendations for reducing infant deaths in the sleep environment. Pediatrics 2022;150(1). e2022057990.

24. Barlow J, Herath NI, Bartram Torrance C, et al. The neonatal behavioral assessment Scale (NBAS) and newborn behavioral observations (NBO) system for supporting caregivers and improving outcomes in caregivers and their infants. Cochrane developmental, psychosocial and learning problems group. Cochrane Database Syst Rev 2018;2018(3). https://doi.org/10.1002/14651858.CD011754.pub2.

25. Bruzek JL, Thompson RH, Witts BN. A review of crying and caregiving: crying as a stimulus. Perspect Behav Sci 2024;47(1):71–105.

26. Tronick E, Beeghly M. Infants' meaning-making and the development of mental health problems. Am Psychol 2011;66(2):107–19.

27. Savage JS. A fourth trimester action plan for wellness. J Perinat Educ 2020;29(2): 103–12.

28. 4th Trimester Project - A Village for Mothers. 4th trimester Project. Available at: https://newmomhealth.com/. Accessed August 1, 2024.

Complementary and Alternative Medicine for Menopause

Melan Javonne Smith-Francis, DNP, CNM, FNP-c*

KEYWORDS

- Menopause • Vasomotor symptoms • Hot flashes
- Complementary and alternative medicine (CAM) • Herbal supplements

KEY POINTS

- Menopause is a natural biological process marking the end of a woman's reproductive years, often accompanied by various symptoms that can significantly impact the quality of life.
- Although hormone replacement therapy (HRT) has been the conventional treatment of menopausal symptoms, concerns about its safety have led many women to seek alternative approaches.
- Complementary and alternative medicine (CAM) has gained popularity with more than 50% of women as a holistic and naturalistic approach to managing menopausal symptoms.
- The National Center for Complementary and Integrative Health (NCCIH) distinguishes between the terms complementary and alternative: when a nonmainstream approach is used alongside conventional medicine it is complementary, whereas when it is used instead of traditional medicine, it is considered alternative.

INTRODUCTION

Menopausal symptoms such as hot flashes, night sweats, mood swings, vaginal dryness, reduced energy, sleep disturbances, and muscle and joint pain can significantly impact women's well-being during the transition to menopause. Menopause generally begins around the age of 51, with the average range being between 40 and 58 years.[1] As an alternative or complement to conventional treatments, complementary and alternative medicine (CAM) provides a varied array of approaches to minimize the changes associated with menopause. This article seeks to critically assess evidence regarding the utilization of CAM for alleviating menopausal symptoms. Complementary and integrative modalities can be classified into 5 domains: biological based,

Midwifery, Bethel University, St Paul, MN, USA
* Corresponding author.
E-mail address: mjs57934@bethel.edu

Nurs Clin N Am 59 (2024) 551–562
https://doi.org/10.1016/j.cnur.2024.08.001   nursing.theclinics.com
0029-6465/24/© 2024 Elsevier Inc. All rights reserved, including those for text and data mining, AI training, and similar technologies.

manipulative based, mind-body based, energy based, and whole system based.[2] This article focuses on the biological domain, which includes supplements, botanicals, nutrition, homeopathy, and aromatherapy for managing menopausal symptoms.

SUPPLEMENTS AND BOTANICALS
Black Cohosh (Cimicifuga racemosa)

Historically, black cohosh has been used to alleviate menopausal symptoms.[3] Recent studies[4,5] have shown conflicting results regarding the efficacy of black cohosh in relieving hot flashes and other menopausal symptoms. Although some trials report significant improvements, others suggest limited benefits. The usual dose of black cohosh for vasomotor symptoms (VMS) is 20 to 40 mg twice a day.[6] However, the most commonly used form is an extract of black cohosh standardized to contain 1 mg of triterpenes, specifically 27-deoxyactein, per tablet, known by the trade name Remifemin. This extract is reported to relieve hot flashes, depression, and vaginal atrophy. In a large study involving 629 female patients, this extract demonstrated significant efficacy, with more than 80% of patients experiencing clear improvement in menopausal symptoms within 6 to 8 weeks. Both physical and psychological symptoms were alleviated with its use.[3,4] A meta-analysis of 9 randomized controlled trials (RCTs) found a significant reduction in the frequency of VMS compared with controls, indicating potential efficacy. However, safety concerns, particularly regarding liver toxicity, warrant careful consideration when recommending black cohosh to menopausal women.[4]

Various literature differ on the length of consumption concerning safety; however, most studies limit consumption to 6 months. Caution is advised when coadministering with antihypertensive agents due to potential potentiation effects. Side effects are rare but may include gastrointestinal upset, headache, dizziness, hypotension, or painful extremities, particularly with higher doses. Furthermore, black cohosh has been associated with liver toxicity, necessitating caution when used concomitantly with statins, cytochrome P450-active drugs, or other hepatotoxic agents.[4,6] Recent research suggests that black cohosh may not possess estrogenic properties, contrary to earlier beliefs. However, its exact mechanisms of action remain unclear. Studies have proposed various hypotheses, including serotonin receptor modulation and antioxidant. Further research is needed to elucidate the precise pathways through which black cohosh affects menopausal symptoms.

Red Clover (Trifolium pratense)

Red clover is a botanic containing isoflavone. Isoflavones are chemical compounds with phytoestrogenic properties. Isoflavones (coumestrol, genistein, and daidzein) are also found in soybeans (highest concentration), clover, chickpeas, and lentils and are considered to be the most potent estrogens among phytoestrogens. These compounds have a chemical structure similar to the estrogen naturally produced by the body, but their effectiveness as estrogen is much lower, estimated to be only 1/1000 to 1/100,000 of that of estradiol, a natural estrogen.[7]

Promensil (in extract form) contains 40 mg of total isoflavones per dose. A meta-analysis of RCTs evaluated its use but found it ineffective in reducing the incidence of VMS. However, a subsequent RCT involving 109 postmenopausal women aged 40 years and older demonstrated some effectiveness for this indication. In this trial, the treatment group received 2 daily capsules containing 80 mg of red clover isoflavones or a matched placebo. The red clover significantly reduced the frequency of hot flashes and the overall intensity of menopausal symptoms.[6]

Some studies suggest that isoflavones, particularly genistein and daidzein, may help relieve hot flashes and other symptoms of menopause.[8] It may take up to 13 weeks for the effects of soy isoflavones to become noticeable.[2] However, it is important to note that whereas some phytoestrogens may have estrogenic effects, others can have antiestrogenic properties. Long-term use of phytoestrogens in postmenopausal women has been associated with endometrial hyperplasia, which can be a precursor to cancer.[9] Therefore, although red clover and other sources of isoflavones may offer benefits for managing menopausal symptoms, their long-term safety, particularly concerning their effects on endometrial health, needs careful consideration.

Evening Primrose Oil (Oenothera biennis)

Evening primrose oil is rich in omega-6 fatty acids and is used for various conditions such as rheumatoid arthritis, atopic dermatitis, and myalgia, as well as symptoms related to menopause and menstruation. Evening primrose is used in divided doses at 3 to 4 g to manage hot flashes and mastalgia.[6] Evening primrose oil has been associated with potential risks, particularly in individuals with seizure disorders, because it may potentiate the risk of seizures. Caution is warranted when using evening primrose oil concomitantly with phenothiazines and other medications that lower the seizure threshold. Common side effects include diarrhea and nausea.[9,10] However, despite its widespread use, evidence regarding the therapeutic benefits of evening primrose oil for the treatment of menopause symptoms remains limited. Only 2 clinical trials investigating its potential efficacy in this context have been conducted, and neither demonstrated significant therapeutic benefits.[6,11,12] Although evening primrose oil holds promise for managing various conditions, including menopause-related symptoms, caution should be exercised due to potential safety concerns, particularly regarding its effect on seizure risk. Further research is warranted to elucidate its mechanisms of action and determine its efficacy and safety profile in managing menopause symptoms.

Dong Quai (Angelica sinensis)

Dong quai is believed to exert its effects through various mechanisms, although the precise mechanism of action still needs to be fully understood. Dong quai is thought to contain compounds that have estrogenic properties, which may help alleviate menopausal symptoms such as hot flashes and vaginal dryness.[13] Dong quai, often used for menopausal symptoms, is typically administered at 3 to 4 g daily, divided into doses. However, due to potential interactions,[2,14] caution is advised when using dong quai concurrently with anticoagulation drugs like warfarin.

Although dong quai may offer benefits for managing menopausal symptoms, caution should be exercised, especially in individuals taking anticoagulation medications. Further research is needed to understand its mechanism of action better and to determine its efficacy and safety profile in menopause management.

Maca (Lepidium meyenii)

Maca is believed to exert its effects through the modulation of hormonal levels, although the precise mechanism of action is not fully elucidated. Maca is hypothesized to act on the hypothalamus and pituitary glands, leading to the regulation of hormone production, which may help alleviate menopause symptoms such as hot flashes and mood swings.[15] Maca, often used for various health purposes, including menopause symptoms, is typically administered at 2 to 4 g daily, divided into doses. However, caution is warranted, especially in individuals with hormone-sensitive cancers, due to potential interactions.[2] Despite its potential benefits, safety concerns exist, particularly regarding its use in individuals with hormone-sensitive cancers. Maca contains compounds that may influence hormone levels, potentially exacerbating hormone-sensitive cancers or interfering with hormone therapy.[16]

St John's Wort (Hypericum perforatum)

St John's wort is widely used for both depression and relief of menopause-related symptoms. Research indicates that St John's wort may improve sleep and enhance menopause-related quality of life; however, it has shown no significant benefit for reducing hot flashes. Often, it is combined with black cohosh to treat menopause symptoms.[17,18] St John's wart is commonly administered at a dosage of 300 mg 3 times daily for the management of VMS, irritability, and depression associated with menopause.[2] The mechanism of action of St John's wort involves its ability to modulate neurotransmitter levels, particularly serotonin, norepinephrine, and dopamine, within the brain. This modulation is believed to contribute to its antidepressant effects.[19]

Despite its potential benefits, St John's wort is associated with safety concerns and numerous drug interactions; it interferes with the metabolism of many medications metabolized in the liver by the cytochrome P450 enzyme system, including estrogen, digoxin, and theophylline. Additionally, it can reduce international normalized ratio levels and should not be used concomitantly with antidepressants such as monoamine oxidase inhibitors (MAOIs) or immunosuppressants. Common side effects of St John's wort include photosensitivity, rash, constipation, cramping, dry mouth, fatigue, dizziness, restlessness, and insomnia.[20] Although St John's wort may offer benefits for managing menopause-related symptoms and depression, caution should be exercised due to its potential for inducing cytochrome P450 and causing severe drug interactions, particularly with medications such as selective serotonin reuptake inhibitors (SSRIs), serotonin and norepinephrine reuptake inhibitors (SNRIs), and benzodiazepines.

The most extensively researched supplements for managing menopause symptoms include black cohosh, red clover, soy isoflavones, and St John's wort. However, women have also explored various other supplements. Although individual results may vary, some women report relief from menopause symptoms with either a single supplement or a combination of them. The upcoming section of this article explores additional methods that have been documented to provide positive outcomes for managing menopause symptoms.

Relizen

Swedish pollen extract, marketed as Relizen, has gained traction in the United States over the past 5 years as a solution for VMS related to menopause. Originating in Europe, where it has been available for more than 15 years, Relizen is derived from flower pollen and is promoted as a nonallergenic option. Despite its European origins, Relizen has undergone scrutiny in several small randomized clinical trials, demonstrating no estrogenic effects or endometrial activity. The mechanism of action is attributed to serotonergic activity, with subpharmacologic levels of phytoestrogens. In a RCT involving 54 women, Relizen exhibited efficacy in reducing VMS, with 65% experiencing improvement compared with 38% in the control group. Typically dosed at 2 tablets per day, Relizen is accessible for purchase online without a prescription.[21,22]

Ginkgo biloba

Ginkgo biloba, derived from the leaves and seeds of the ancient ginkgo tree, is commonly used for cognitive enhancement and memory improvement.[23] The typical recommended dosage ranges from 40 to 80 mg orally 3 times daily. Although research suggests its efficacy in enhancing mental flexibility, studies have shown no significant difference compared with placebo in alleviating mood disorders, sleep disturbances, menopause-related symptoms, memory enhancement, or sustained attention.[14] Memory changes, often associated with sleep disturbances, may benefit from ginkgo supplementation. Menopausal sleep disturbances, frequently linked to VMS or other stressors, may also find relief through ginkgo use.

However, like any supplement, ginkgo is not without side effects. Common adverse effects include gastrointestinal distress and hypotension. Chronic use has been associated with more severe complications such as subarachnoid hemorrhage, subdural hematoma, and increased bleeding times. These risks highlight the importance of cautious and informed use, especially in individuals with preexisting health conditions or those taking medications that may interact with ginkgo.

Ginkgo biloba may improve mental flexibility; its efficacy for other conditions remains inconclusive. Furthermore, users should be aware of the possible side effects and risks associated with chronic use, emphasizing the necessity for informed decision making and close monitoring when incorporating ginkgo into one's health care regimen.[6,24,25]

Ginseng

Ginseng, derived from the root of the *Panax ginseng* plant, has been traditionally used in Chinese medicine for its purported benefits on mental acuity and general health. The active compounds in ginseng, known as ginsenosides or panaxoside, contribute to its pharmacologic effects, although the exact mechanism of action remains unclear.[6,23] Commonly consumed as a brewed tea or in pill form, Chinese ginseng is native to Asia and has historically been taken to enhance mental function.[23] It is thought to exert estrogenlike effects in the body, which can be beneficial for some conditions but contraindicated in others, such as breast cancer. Moreover, caution is advised when taking ginseng concurrently with MAOIs, certain depression medications, or anticoagulants, because it may potentiate their effects.

The recommended dosage of *Panax ginseng* typically ranges from 1 to 2 g of root orally daily, divided into doses. This dosage is often used as a general tonic to improve mood, alleviate fatigue, increase energy levels, and address menopause-related symptoms and sexual dysfunction. Although research has shown mixed results regarding its efficacy in managing menopausal symptoms, some studies suggest benefits for overall well-being, general health, and depression.

Despite its potential benefits, ginseng is not without risks. Adverse effects may include dry mouth, rapid heartbeat, nausea, vomiting, diarrhea, insomnia, and nervousness. Additionally, ginseng has been associated with uterine bleeding and mastalgia, particularly in women with breast cancer, highlighting the importance of careful consideration before use.

Ginseng's role as an adaptogen or tonic herb is attributed to its ability to stimulate the hypothalamus-pituitary-adrenal axis, supporting the body during stress and bolstering the immune system. Gingseng's promotion for mood and cognition improvement during menopause underscores its perceived benefits in addressing this population's hormonal changes and cognitive function.

Although ginseng holds promise as a natural remedy for various health concerns, including menopause-related symptoms, its use should be approached cautiously due to potential interactions and adverse effects. Clinicians and individuals considering ginseng supplementation should weigh its potential benefits against its associated risks, especially in populations with specific health conditions or medication regimens.[26,27]

Kava (Piper methysticum)

Kava has been traditionally used for its sedative and analgesic effects. Kava is commonly used to alleviate irritability and insomnia, with research supporting its efficacy in reducing anxiety. One study indicated a decrease in hot flashes, anxiety, and depression, alongside improvements in well-being, whereas another study showed no significant difference.[28] The recommended dosage typically ranges from 150 to 300 mg of root extract orally daily, divided into doses.[6] The mechanism of action of Kava remains incompletely understood; however, it is thought to involve modulation of neurotransmitter activity, particularly gamma-aminobutyric acid receptors, resulting in its anxiolytic effects. Despite its potential benefits, Kava has been banned in several countries due to reports of hepatotoxicity, prompting caution and discouragement of its use. Notably, Kava is contraindicated in individuals with depression due to concerns about exacerbating symptoms. Common side effects associated with Kava consumption include gastrointestinal discomfort, impaired reflexes and motor function, weight loss, and hepatotoxicity.[29] Given the severe risks of liver damage associated with Kava use, its use is not recommended, and individuals considering its use should be informed about these potential adverse effects. Kava may offer some benefits for anxiety and related symptoms, but its potential for hepatotoxicity outweighs its therapeutic potential. Clinicians and individuals exploring CAM options should exercise caution and prioritize safer alternatives for managing anxiety and insomnia.

Sage (Salvia officinalis)

Garden sage is rightly named "salvia," meaning the savior, for its reputed ability to alleviate menopause-related sweating and hot flashes, with noticeable effects within 2 hours. Sage is also claimed to alleviate depression. Recommended dosages include 1 to 2 teaspoons of dried leaf infusion, taken 1 to 8 times daily, or 15 to 40 drops of fresh leaf tincture, administered 1 to 3 times a week.[30,31] Sage has demonstrated promising results in alleviating menopausal symptoms. In a recent open multicenter RCT, a once-daily tablet of sage leaves taken for 8 weeks significantly reduced the intensity and frequency of hot flashes, accompanied by a notable 43% decrease in menopause rating scale scores.[32] However, caution is warranted regarding sage leaf and essential oil consumption, because large amounts or prolonged exposure may lead to adverse effects such as restlessness, vomiting, tachycardia, and seizures. This toxicity is attributed to the presence of camphor and thujone. A dose equivalent to 12 drops of sage essential oil or 15 g of sage leaves can induce toxic effects.[33]

Hops (Humulus lupulus)

Hops have emerged as a potential remedy for menopausal symptoms. Whether consumed orally as dried herb or applied topically as a gel containing 100 μg of 8-prenylnaringenin, hops have shown efficacy in alleviating a spectrum of menopausal issues, including hot flashes, sweats, palpitations, irritability, insomnia, and even water retention.[14,30] Traditionally recognized for their mild hypnotic properties to promote sleep and manage sleep disturbances, headaches, and gynecologic disorders, hops have garnered attention for their estrogen-producing effects. Additionally, hops can be consumed as tea made from dried flowers or as a tincture, typically 5 to 15 drops once or twice daily. Hops also offer a source of B vitamins, adding to their potential nutritional benefits.[30,34]

Vitamin E

Vitamin E, a fat-soluble antioxidant, has been suggested to benefit menopausal symptoms, although evidence remains limited. Anecdotal accounts highlight its potential, yet few RCTs have investigated its efficacy.

In a crossover trial involving 120 women, administration of 800 IU of vitamin E resulted in a reported decrease of 1 hot flash per day, which the authors deemed clinically insignificant.[35] Similarly, another randomized crossover trial with 50 women taking 400 IU of vitamin E demonstrated a reduction of about 2 hot flashes per day and decreased severity.[36,37] Additionally, in an RCT comparing gabapentin to vitamin E for reduction of VMS, vitamin E showed a modest decrease in hot flash frequency and severity.[38] Although some individuals may experience relief from mild hot flashes, scientific evidence supporting the effectiveness of vitamin E remains lacking. Moreover, caution is advised regarding dosing, because higher doses, such as 400 IU, may pose cardiovascular disease risks.[38]

AROMATHERAPY

Aromatherapy, or essential oil therapy, harnesses aromatic essences derived from plants to address a range of physiologic and psychological imbalances. These fragrant oils can alleviate anxiety, induce relaxation, and potentially alleviate stressful menopausal symptoms. In a study by Chien and colleagues,[39] inhalation of lavender for 12 weeks improved self-reported sleep compared with a health education control group. Additionally, a double-blind 12-week clinical crossover trial involving 100 women revealed that lavender essential oil significantly reduced hot flash frequency by 50% compared with a placebo control.[40] This finding demonstrated a clinically significant difference in symptom reduction. Further research, including 3 RCTs combining aromatherapy with massage, indicated that aromatherapy massage was more effective than massage alone or control interventions in reducing both physical symptoms such as VMS and psychological symptoms like depression.[41] Aromatic and topical use of essential oils such as clary sage (*Salvia sclarea*), fennel (*Foeniculum vulgare*), and wild orange (*Citrus sinensis*) are widespread and offer beneficial effects in alleviating menopausal symptoms and scorching flashes.[42]

The incorporation of aromatherapy into other (CAM) interventions may offer additional relief for menopausal symptoms. However, current evidence suggests that aromatherapy alone may not be sufficient as a stand-alone treatment for managing menopausal symptoms.

In addition to lavender, peppermint oil is another beneficial essential oil. Diluted peppermint oil applied to the feet has been reported to provide cooling relief, which may help alleviate hot flashes and discomfort associated with menopause.[43]

HOMEOPATHIC

Sepia officinalis, extracted from the inky juice of cuttlefish, and China rubra (*Arenaria rubra* or *China officinalis*) are homeopathic remedies for managing menopausal symptoms. For *S officinalis*, the recommended dosage is 30C, with 5 pellets dissolved sublingually in the morning and evening.[44,45] For China rubra, the suggested dosage is 9C, involving the dissolution of 5 pellets sublingually each morning for 10 to 14 days. Noticeable improvements in moodiness and sensitivity have been reported after 3 doses.[45,46]

NUTRITION

Phytoestrogen-containing foods, such as soy, flaxseed, nuts, whole grains, and certain vegetables, contain plant compounds that can interact with estrogen receptors in the body. These foods are commonly found in plant-based diets and are associated with various health benefits. High intake of phytoestrogen-rich foods has been linked to a reduction in menopausal symptoms, including hot flashes, as well as an increase in mature vaginal cells, which can alleviate vaginal dryness and irritation. Additionally, phytoestrogens have been shown to inhibit osteoporosis and decrease the risk of breast, colon, and prostate cancers. Despite exerting estrogenic effects, phytoestrogens are considered to be much weaker than endogenous estrogens, with only about 2% of their activity. Soy, in particular, has been studied extensively for its potential to relieve hot flashes and atrophic vaginitis. Research suggests that consuming enough soy to provide approximately 200 mg of isoflavones can lead to signs of estrogenic activity, such as an increase in vaginal superficial cells. This effect helps counteract the vaginal dryness and irritation often experienced during menopause.[3,47,48]

Flaxseeds are a nutritional powerhouse, rich in omega-3 fatty acids, magnesium, potassium, and fiber. Although omega-3 fatty acids are readily available from fish, alternatives like flaxseeds provide a plant-based source. In Japan, where seaweed and soy foods are commonly consumed, only 10% to 20% of women experience hot flashes, in contrast to the 70% to 80% prevalence in Western countries. Studies have shown that soy protein containing 60 mg of isoflavones can significantly reduce hot flashes by 57% and night sweats by 43%.

To mitigate menopausal symptoms, adopting a diet comprising 50% raw foods and incorporating a protein supplement can help stabilize blood sugar levels. Including foods such as blackstrap molasses, soybean products, broccoli, dandelion greens, kelp, salmon with bones, sardines, and whitefish can further enhance nutritional intake. Limiting dairy products to yogurt or buttermilk is advisable, because dairy and meat consumption has been linked to increased hot flashes. Additionally, avoiding alcohol, caffeine, sugar, spicy foods, and hot soups/drinks can help prevent triggering hot flashes and aggravating urinary incontinence and mood swings. These substances can also acidify the blood, releasing calcium from bones and contributing to bone loss. Adequate hydration, achieved by consuming 2 quarts of quality water daily, is crucial for preventing dry skin and mucous membranes.[3,48,49]

SUMMARY

Although the evidence supporting the use of CAM for menopause is promising, further research is needed to establish the long-term efficacy and safety of these approaches. The use of CAM among peri- and menopausal women is widespread, with studies indicating that up to 91% of women report its utilization.[6] Women turn to CAM for various reasons, including symptom management, perceived naturalness, fewer side effects compared with prescriptions, and the belief that it promotes overall health and quality of life. Additionally, recommendations from family, friends, or clinicians and the desire for disease prevention contribute to its popularity. However, many women neglect to disclose their CAM use to clinicians because of negative past experiences.

Given the substantial number of women using CAM and the apparent lack of disclosure to clinicians, health care providers must familiarize themselves with various CAM modalities and engage in open discussions with women about their usage. However, the efficacy and safety of CAM still needs to be researched, primarily due to the need for more high-quality studies. Existing research often needs to improve on limitations such as small sample sizes, lack of control groups, and short durations, which hinder clinicians' ability to make informed recommendations.

Addressing these gaps in knowledge and understanding is crucial to providing comprehensive care to peri- and menopausal women. Clinicians should advocate for increased research funding and rigorous study designs to evaluate the effectiveness and safety of CAM therapies, ensuring that women receive evidence-based guidance to make informed decisions about their health and well-being.[50,51] Integrating CAM into menopausal care requires a personalized approach, considering individual preferences, health status, and cultural factors. Health care providers should engage in open and informed discussions with menopausal women, weighing CAM modalities' benefits and potential risks.

CLINICS CARE POINTS

- Evidence supports a personalized approach to the management of menopause.
- Engaging in open, informed discussions with patients about CAM options, their efficacy, and safety is essential.
- Some CAM therapies, such as acupuncture and mindfulness are timeless however other treatments have minimal to moderate evidence supporting their use in reducing vasomotor symptoms and improving quality of life in menopausal women.
- Clinicians must exercise caution when prescribing CAM modalities due to poor regulation.
- Clinical should continuously assess for side effects and closely monitor their patients who initiate CAM treatments.
- While some CAM therapies show promise, there is still a lack of research, in particular randomized control trials. Without methods to reduce bias, recommending certain CAM treatments remains speculative.

DISCLOSURE

I, M.J. Smith-Francis, hereby affirm that I have no commercial or financial conflicts of interest to declare relevant to the subject matter discussed herein.

REFERENCES

1. North American Menopause Society. Are we there yet? navigate now with our guided menopause tour. Menopause.org 2024. Available at: https://www.menopause.org/for-women/menopauseflashes/menopause-symptoms-and-treatments/are-we-there-yet-navigate-now-with-our-guided-menopause-tour. Accessed July 17, 2024.
2. Barbieri A, Fenske S. Complementary and integrative approaches in obstetrics and gynecology. Clinical Updates Women's Health Care 2021;XX(4):1–48.
3. Murray M, Pizzorno J. Menopause. In: Murray M, Pizzorno J, editors. Encyclopedia of natural medicine. 2nd edition. Rocklin, CA: Prima Publishing; 1998. p. 629–644.1.
4. Smith IE, Williamson EM, Putnam S, et al. Black Cohosh (Actaea racemosa) in menopause – is it safe? a systematic review and meta-analysis. Maturitas 2020;136:57–67.

5. Shams T, Setia MS, Hemmings R, et al. Efficacy of black Cohosh-containing preparations on menopausal symptoms: a meta-analysis. Alternative Ther Health Med 2020;26(2):32–40.

6. Bruckner MC, King TL. Pharmacology for women's health. 2nd edition. Burlington, MA: Jones & Bartlett Learning; 2017.

7. Setchell KDR, Brown NM, Lydeking-Olsen E. The clinical importance of the metabolite equol-a clue to the effectiveness of soy and its isoflavones. J Nutr 2002;132(12):3577–84.

8. Tempfer CB, Bentz EK, Leodolter S, et al. Phytoestrogens in clinical practice: a review of the literature. Fertil Steril 2007;87(6):1243–9.

9. Atkinson C, Warren RM, Sala E, et al. Red clover-derived isoflavones and mammographic breast density: a double-blind, randomized, placebo-controlled trial [ISRCTN42940165]. Breast Cancer Res 2004;6(3):R170–9.

10. Farzaneh F, Fatehi S, Sohrabi MR, et al. The effect of oral evening primrose oil on menopausal hot flashes: a randomized clinical trial. Arch Gynecol Obstet 2013; 288(5):1075–9.

11. Chenoy R, Hussain S, Tayob Y, et al. Effect of oral gamolenic acid from evening primrose oil on menopausal flushing. BMJ 1994;308(6927):501–3.

12. Setchell KD, Borriello SP, Hulme P, et al. Nonsteroidal estrogens of dietary origin: possible roles in hormone-dependent disease. Am J Clin Nutr 1984;40(3): 569–78.

13. Haines CJ, Lam PM, Chung TK, et al. A randomized, double-blind, placebo-controlled study of the effect of a Chinese herbal medicine preparation (Dang Gui Buxue Tang) on menopausal symptoms in Hong Kong Chinese women. Climacteric 2008;11(3):244–51.

14. Tharpe NL, Farley CL, Jordan RG. Clinical practice guidelines for midwifery & women's health. 6th edition. Burlington, MA: Jones & Bartlett Learning; 2022.

15. Meissner HO, Reich-Bilinska H, Mscisz A, et al. Therapeutic effects of pregelatinized maca (Lepidium peruvianum Chacon) used as a non-hormonal alternative to HRT in perimenopausal women - clinical pilot study. Int J Biomed Sci 2006;2(2):143–59.

16. Gonzales GF, Gonzales-Castañeda C. The use of maca (Lepidium meyenii) to improve semen quality: A systematic review. Maturitas 2018;116:6–10.

17. Uebelhack R, Blohmer JU, Graubaum HJ, et al. Black cohosh and St. John's wort for climacteric complaints: a randomized trial. Obstet Gynecol 2006;107(2 Pt 1): 247–55.

18. van Die MD, Burger HG, Teede HJ, et al. Vitex agnus-castus extracts for female reproductive disorders: a systematic review of clinical trials. Planta Med 2013; 79(7):562–75.

19. Butterweck V. Mechanism of action of St John's wort in depression: what is known? CNS Drugs 2003;17(8):539–62.

20. Markowitz JS, Donovan JL, DeVane CL, et al. Effect of St. John's wort on drug metabolism by induction of cytochrome P450 3A4 enzyme. JAMA 2003; 290(11):1500–4.

21. Secor RM, Holland AC, Carcio HA. Advanced health assessment of women: skills, procedures, and management. 5th ediiton. New York, NY: Springer Publishing; 2024.

22. Stute P, Nisslein T, Meier B, et al. Efficacy and safety of the special extract ERr 731 from the roots of rheum rhaponticum in perimenopausal women with menopausal symptoms. Menopause 2006;13(5):744–59.

23. Minkin MJ, Wright CV. A woman's guide to menopause & perimenopause. New Haven, CT: Yale University Press Health & Wellness; 2005.

24. Mix JA, Crews WD Jr. An examination of the efficacy of Ginkgo biloba extract EGb761 on the neuropsychologic functioning of cognitively intact older adults. J Alternative Compl Med 2000;6(3):219–29.

25. Yuan QL, Wang P, Liu L, et al. Ginkgo biloba for mild cognitive impairment and Alzheimer's disease: a systematic review and meta-analysis of randomized controlled trials. Curr Top Med Chem 2016;16(5):520–8. https://doi.org/10.2174/1568026615666150825115607.

26. Kennedy DO, Scholey AB. Ginseng: potential for the enhancement of cognitive performance and mood. Pharmacol Biochem Behav 2003;75(3):687–700. https://doi.org/10.1016/s0091-3057(03)00126-6.

27. Yuan CS, Wang CZ, Wicks SM, et al. Chemical and pharmacological studies of saponins with a focus on American ginseng. J Ginseng Res 2010;34(3):160–7. https://doi.org/10.5142/jgr.2010.34.3.160.

28. Pittler MH, Ernst E. Efficacy of kava extract for treating anxiety: systematic review and meta-analysis. J Clin Psychopharmacol 2000;20(1):84–9. https://doi.org/10.1097/00004714-200002000-00016.

29. National Institutes of Health. National Center for Complementary and Integrative Health. Kava. Available at: https://www.nccih.nih.gov/health/kava. Accessed January 25, 2022.

30. Weed SS. Wise woman ways: menopausal years. Woodstock, NY: Ash Tree Publishing; 1992.

31. Garg G, Adams JD. Garden sage (Salvia officinalis) for menopausal hot flushes: Anything new on the horizon? Complement. Ther Med 2019;47:102235. https://doi.org/10.1016/j.ctim.2019.02.005.

32. Bommer S, Klein P, Suter A. First time proof of sage's tolerability and efficacy in menopausal women with hot flushes. Adv Ther 2011;28(6):490–500. https://doi.org/10.1007/s12325-011-0027-z.

33. Adibhatla RM, Hatcher JF. Altered lipid metabolism in brain injury and disorders. Subcell Biochem 2008;49:241–68. https://doi.org/10.1007/978-1-4020-8831-5_8.

34. Johnson R. Hops. In: Coates PM, Betz JM, Blackman MR, et al, editors. Encyclopedia of dietary supplements. 2nd edition. Boca Raton, FL: CRC Press; 2010. https://doi.org/10.1201/b10184-73.

35. Dennehy C, Tsourounis C, Horn AJ. Dietary supplements in women's health: vitamin E. J Pharm Pract 2003;16(3):275–82. https://doi.org/10.1177/089719000301600309.

36. Kronenberg F, Fugh-Berman A. Complementary and alternative medicine for menopausal symptoms: a review of randomized, controlled trials. Ann Intern Med 2002;137(10):805–13. https://doi.org/10.7326/0003-4819-137-10-200211190-00009.

37. MedicineNet.com. Menopause (perimenopause) symptoms and treatments. Available at: http://www.medicinenet.com/script/main/art.asp?articlekey=2036. Accessed November 1, 2010.

38. Hersh EV, Moore PA. Vitamin E and benign oral mucosal lesions. An evaluation. J Am Dent Assoc 1979;99(5):798–800. https://doi.org/10.14219/jada.archive.1979.0005.

39. Chien LW, Cheng SL, Liu CF. The effect of lavender aromatherapy on autonomic nervous system in midlife women with insomnia. Evid Based Complement Alternat Med 2012;2012:740813.

40. Cho HJ, Min SY, Shin MH, et al. Lavender essential oil inhalation reduces nocturnal hot flashes in menopausal women: A randomized controlled trial. Menopause 2017;24(9):1024–31.

41. Hur MH, Lee MS, Seong KY, et al. Aromatherapy massage on the abdomen for alleviating menstrual pain in high school girls: A preliminary controlled clinical study. Evid Based Complement Alternat Med 2012;2012:187163.

42. MacDonald D. The Essential Life: A Simple Guide to Living the Wellness Lifestyle. UT, USA: Total Wellness Publishing; 2015.

43. Nikjou R, Noori M, Maleki-Dizaji S, et al. Peppermint oil effect on nausea and vomiting after open and laparoscopic nephrectomies: A randomized clinical trial. Anesthesiol Pain Med 2016;6(6):e40223. https://doi.org/10.5812/aapm.40223.

44. Ullman D. Homeopathic medicine for women. New York, NY: TarcherPerigee; 1999.

45. Tinney A, Rice E. Homeopathy: a state of the science review with recommendations for practical therapies in midwifery practice. J Midwifery Wom Health 2023; 68(Number S1). Silver Spring, MD.

46. Lockie A, Geddes N. The complete guide to homeopathy: the principles and practice of treatment. London, UK: DK; 2019.

47. Messina M. Soy and health update: evaluation of the clinical and epidemiologic literature. Nutrients 2016;8(12):754.

48. Balch PA. Prescription for nutritional healing: a practical A-to-Z reference to drug-free remedies using vitamins, minerals. In: Bell S, editor. Food supplements. 6th edition. New York, NY: Avery Books; 2023.

49. Northrup C. The wisdom of menopause: creating physical and emotional health during the change. Revised Edition. New York, NY: Bantam Books; 2006.

50. Adams J, Lui CW, Sibbritt D, et al. Women's use of complementary and alternative medicine during pregnancy: a critical review of the literature. Birth 2009;36(3): 237–45. https://doi.org/10.1111/j.1523-536X.2009.00322.x.

51. National Center for Complementary and Integrative Health. Complementary, alternative, or integrative health: what's in a name?. Available at: https://www.nccih.nih.gov/health/complementary-alternative-or-integrative-health-whats-in-a-name. Accessed January 25, 2022.

Best Practices for Identifying and Supporting Patients who Present with PCOS

Angelika Gabrielski, MSN, FNP-C, APRN[a],*,
Shivon Latice Daniels, MSN, FNP-C, APRN[a], Kelsey Frey, MPAS, PA-C[b],
Anica Land, MSN, AGNP-C, APRN[b]

KEYWORDS

- Polycystic ovary syndrome • Menstrual irregularities • Insulin resistance
- Hyperandrogenism • Screening • Diagnosis • Treatment

KEY POINTS

- Polycystic ovary syndrome (PCOS) is a heterogenous familial condition with reproductive, metabolic, and psychologic attributes.
- PCOS is complex, not well-understood, or unrecognized, which can lead to delays in diagnosing and treatment.
- Women with PCOS are at higher risk for developing type 2 diabetes, obesity, cardiovascular complications, hypertension, dyslipidemia, non-alcoholic fatty liver disease, depression, anxiety, and sub-fertility.
- Insulin resistance is a major contributor to onset of cardiovascular, metabolic, and reproductive complications in women with PCOS.
- A multidisciplinary team approach to caring and supporting women with PCOS offers the best path to addressing and meeting the care needs in this population.

INTRODUCTION

Polycystic ovary syndrome (POCS) represents the most common endocrinopathy among reproductive aged women.[1–3] It is a familial heterogenous condition with reproductive, metabolic, and psychologic consequences that typically manifests in adolescence.[1,4,5] Physical features of PCOS include amenorrhea, hirsutism, acne, and associated finding of polycystic ovaries.[5] Prominent features are weight gain and mood swings.[6] PCOS is complex and often underdiagnosed and underreported.[6,7] The time of diagnosis exceeds 2 y on average and can involve 3 or more

[a] Division of Endocrinology, Metabolism and Nutrition, Duke University, 40 Duke Medicine Circle, Durham, NC 27710, USA; [b] Division of Endocrinology, Duke University, 40 Duke Medicine Circle, Durham, NC 27710, USA
* Corresponding author. 10207 Cerny Street, Suite 306, Raleigh, NC 27617.
E-mail address: Angelika.gabrielski@duke.edu

Nurs Clin N Am 59 (2024) 563–575
https://doi.org/10.1016/j.cnur.2024.08.007
0029-6465/24/© 2024 Elsevier Inc. All rights reserved, including those for text and data mining, AI training, and similar technologies.

providers.[7] Protracted diagnosis increases both patient frustration and the risk of PCOS associated co-morbidities, including infertility, depression and anxiety, pregnancy complications, type 2 diabetes (T2DM), endometrial cancer, and cardiovascular disease.[3,5–7]

EPIDEMIOLOGY

PCOS affects 4% to 20% of reproductive aged women depending which criteria is used.[6] According to the World Health Organization, it is estimated that approximately 116 million women world-wide are impacted by PCOS.[6] Acne and hirsutism are prominent features in adolescents, whereas metabolic features are more of a concern later in life. PCOS is a complex, inherited disorder, with an interplay between environmental factors (diet, lifestyle) and genetics.[8] Possible epigenetic initiators include diabetes, fetal exposure to excess androgens and chemicals in the environment, and premature fetal development associated with hypertension.[4,8] Overweight women with family history of PCOS or T2DM are at higher risk of developing PCOS.[4]

PATHOPHYSIOLOGY

Despite the awareness of genetic predisposition for PCOS, the pathophysiology of PCOS is not well-understood. Insulin resistance is one of the key components of PCOS. Insulin resistance leads to hyperinsulinemia,[3] with a consequential decrease in sex hormone binding globulin (SHBG) production by the liver. The result is higher androgen production by the ovary, increased free testosterone in the blood, and an increase in androgenic activity.[3,9]

At the hypothalamic-pituitary level, gonadotropin-releasing hormone (GnRH) pulsation frequency is increased, resulting in a corresponding increase in the secretion of luteinizing hormone (LH).[3,9,10] The LH/follicular stimulating hormone (FSH) ratio also increases. Higher levels of LH stimulate androgen secretion from the ovarian theca cells. Ovarian follicles become resistant to the effects of FSH due to high LH levels during the cycle.[2,4,10] Resistance of the follicles to FSH is what contributes to the polycystic morphology (PCOM) of the ovary. These follicles represent arrested or immature follicles. The end result is menstrual irregularities (oligo- or anovulation, sub-infertility) associated with PCOS.[3,9] Thus, these changes in the hypothalamic-pituitary axis, combined with hyperinsulinemia, contribute to the characteristic manifestations of PCOS.

DIAGNOSIS

In 1990, the National Institutes of Health (NIH) defined PCOS as oligomenorrhea or anovulation *and* evidence of physical and/or biochemical androgen excess.[5] The Rotterdam Criteria, developed in 2003 by the European Society of Human Reproduction and the American Society of Reproductive Medicine, expanded the diagnostic criteria set forth by the NIH to include PCOM on ultrasound.[3] The Rotterdam criteria requires 2 out of 3 of the following features for diagnosis of PCOS: oligomenorrhea or anovulation, clinical and/or biochemical hyperandrogenism, and polycystic ovaries. Yet another diagnostic criterion is offered by the Androgen Excess and PCOS Society, created in 2008.[11–13] The Rotterdam criteria is the most widely used diagnostic criteria[14] and requires that alternative causes of hyperandrogenism are ruled out before confirming a diagnosis of POCS. **Table 1** outlines approaches to diagnosing PCOS. **Table 2** outlines phenotypes.

PCOS is a diagnosis of exclusion as there are other conditions that present with similar symptoms/features.[11] Those conditions include thyroid disease, prolactinoma,

Table 1
Approaches to diagnose polycystic ovary syndrome[3,11–13,15]

Approach	Criteria for Diagnosis		Testing
NIH	Hyperandrogenism Oligomenorrhea		Testosterone level
Rotterdam Criteria	2 of the following:	1. Hyperandrogenism 2. Oligomenorrhea 3. >12 follicles in each ovary or increased ovarian volume of >10 mL	Ovarian ultrasound
AES	Biochemical or clinical hyperandrogenism with 1 of the following:	1. Oligomenorrhea with follicles on ovaries 2. Follicles on ovaries without oligomenorrhea	Ovarian ultrasound Total testosterone

androgen-producing tumors, non-classical adrenal hyperplasia, primary ovarian insufficiency, and LH hormone hypersecretion.[11–13] Comorbid screening laboratories for prediabetes, T2DM, hyperlipidemia, and liver dysfunction should be conducted.[22,23] Hormonal contraception can lower free and total testosterone; patients should be counseled to discontinue use for at least 3 mo prior to testing. High quality assay is recommended when checking total and free testosterone level. Biotin supplements can interfere with thyroid assay; patients should be counseled to discontinue biotin supplements prior to thyroid function assessed. **Table 3** provides an overview of recommended laboratory tests.

Clinical presentation may prompt consideration of additional laboratory tests. Clinical indicators of PCOS include acne, hirsutism, male pattern hair loss, subfertility, and menstrual irregularities.[3,10] **Table 4** outlines key definitions.[14,18] Comprehensive physical examination, exploration of chief concerns, and detailed patient history (current medications, personal history, date of last menstrual cycle, family history, and social history) round out the initial assessment.[12]

Elevated total testosterone, free testosterone, androstenedione, and dehydroepiandrosterone sulfate can be associated with hyperandrogenism.[12] Clinical features of hyperandrogenism include female hirsutism, male pattern baldness, and/or cystic acne.[18] The Ferriman-Gallwey scoring system is an available tool used to evaluate the level and severity of hirsutism.[18] For patients with hyperandrogenism and oligoanovulation, non-classic adrenal hyperplasia should be ruled out. Patients with

Table 2
Rotterdam phenotypes[14,16–21]

Phenotype	Criteria
A	1. Hyperandrogenism 2. Oligo-anovulation 3. Polycystic ovarian morphology on ultrasound
B	1. Hyperandrogenism 2. Oligo-anovulation
C	1. Hyperandrogenism 2. Polycystic ovarian morphology on ultrasound
D	1. Oligo-anovulation 2. Polycystic ovarian morphology on ultrasound

Table 3
Diagnostic testing[11–13,22,23]

Test Name	Indication	Test Interpretation
Beta Human Chorionic Gonadotropin (HCG)	Screen for pregnancy	Positive result confirms pregnancy
Thyroid Stimulating Hormone (TSH)	Screen for thyroid dysfunction	High or Low value confirms thyroid dysfunction
Luteinizing Hormone (LH)	Screen for LH hypersecretion	Elevated LH in PCOS
Follicular-Stimulating Hormone (FSH)	Screen for primary ovarian failure	Normal or low FSH in PCOS
Prolactin	Hyperprolactinemia	Elevation may be due to a prolactin secreting pituitary tumor
Testosterone Total	Screen for androgen secreting tumor	Mild elevation may be due to PCOS
Testosterone Free	Screen for biochemical hyperandrogenism	Mild/higher levels in PCOS
Dehydroepiandrosterone-sulfate (DHEA-S)	To rule out an androgen secreting tumor	Mild elevation may be due to PCOS
Hemoglobin A1c 2-h 75-g OGTT Fasting insulin/glucose	Screen for prediabetes/T2DM Screen for impaired glucose intolerance, T2DM Screen for insulin resistance.	Co-morbid screening
17-Hydroxyprogesterone	Screen for nonclassical congenital adrenal hyperplasia	Elevation confirms non- classical congenital adrenal hyperplasia
Pelvic or Transvaginal Ultrasound	Assess for PCOM	>12 follicles, 2–9 mm in diameter in each ovary with a string of pearl morphology, or increased ovarian volume of >10 mL
Liver function	Baseline liver function	Co-morbid screen for NAFLD
Lipid Panel	Screen for hypercholesteremia	Low HDL, high LDL cholesterol levels, & high triglycerides confirm hypercholesteremia

Table 4 Definitions[14,18]	
Metabolic Syndrome	Characterized by Obesity, Hypertension, Dyslipidemia, and Hyperglycemia
Female Hirsutism	Excessive terminal hair growth in a male pattern
Androgenic pattern alopecia	Hair loss/thinning beginning at the part line
Polycystic Ovary Morphology (PCOM)	Enlarged ovaries with small peripheral cysts and increased stroma
Oligomenorrhea	Irregular menstrual cycles with a skip of 3 or more cycles
Hyperandrogenism	A condition with elevated androgen levels characterized by acne, oily skin, male pattern baldness, and excessive hair on the face, chest, and stomach

amenorrhea should have tests for prolactin, FSH, and thyroid stimulating hormone to rule out prolactinoma, thyroid disease, and primary ovarian insufficiency.[12,14]

PCOS is associated with significant morbidities, which include obesity, insulin resistance, nonalcoholic fatty liver (NAFLD), T2DM, metabolic syndrome, cardiovascular disease, hypertension, dyslipidemia, sleep disorders (obstructive sleep apnea [OSA]), adverse pregnancy outcomes (pre-term birth, gestational diabetes, delivery by cesarean section, pre-eclampsia, small term birth, and birth defects), mood disorders (depression, anxiety), and uterine cancer.[2,10,24,25]

Obesity is more severe in phenotype A.[10] Obesity increases insulin resistance, which increases risk of fatty liver. More than half of women with PCOS have insulin resistance.[2,10] Insulin resistance promotes androgen production and lowers SHBG, which leads to inflammation and the deposition of fat in the liver. Obesity, insulin resistance, and metabolic syndrome contribute to the development of NAFLD.[2,10]

Women with PCOS carry a higher risk of developing T2DM compared to the normal population. Body mass index (BMI) greater than 25 is a risk factor for development of T2DM. There are higher rates of glucose intolerance in obese women with PCOS.[5,8,10]

Women with PCOS have a higher incidence of metabolic syndrome characterized by low protective high-density lipoprotein,[12] higher triglycerides, higher waist circumference, and higher rate of abnormal oral glucose tolerance test results. Women with PCOS have higher rates of cardiovascular disease associated with hypertension and hyperlipidemia.[19,26,27]

Women with PCOS have a higher risk for sleep disturbances and OSA.[3]

Women with PCOS have a higher rate of depression, with likely contributing factors of irregular periods, infertility, physical effects of hyperandrogenism (acne, hirsutism), body image distress, and delays in diagnosis and treatment.[3,10,18]

Women with PCOS have a higher rate of uterine cancer associated with chronic unopposed estrogen. Chronic anovulation leads to endometrial hyperplasia, compounded by obesity and insulin resistance. This is seen frequently in pre-menopausal women.[5,14,15,18]

POLYCYSTIC OVARY SYNDROME TREATMENT

Treatment for PCOS is focused on addressing the physical, metabolic, and psychologic effects of hyperandrogenism and chronic anovulation.[28] Given the complexity of care required, a multi-disciplinary team approach should be considered and include endocrinology, gynecology, dermatology, gastroenterology, sleep specialist, and registered dietician/nutritionist. It is important to note that most of the treatment modalities listed are off-label.

HYPERANDROGENISM

Hirsutism, acne, and androgen-related alopecia are visible features of hyperandrogenism and can be very distressing. Treatments include combination oral contraceptive pill (COCP), androgen blockers, and topical preparations that address these conditions.[24]

The first line treatment for hirsutism is COCP.[3,10,24] COCP suppresses gonadotropin section and ovarian androgen production. Medication with progestin with lower androgenic activity is optimal. However, providers should consider risk for venous thrombosis (VTE) and personal history when making selection. Spironolactone is an androgen receptor blocker (decreases ovarian testosterone production) and inhibits 5 alpha reductase activity.[10,29] Spironolactone can be added after 6 mo of treatment with COCP to address hirsutism. Start with 50 mg twice daily with option to titrate up to max daily dose of 100 mg twice daily. This is a teratogen; reliable birth control required. Other considerations include monitoring blood pressure and potassium. Topical eflornithine addresses hirsutism (facial hair) but may worsen acne. It works by inhibiting enzyme activity that stimulates growth and development of hair follicles. Flutamide (androgen blocker) is another option, but reliable birth control is required due to possible teratogenic effects. Liver function should be monitored before initiation of therapy, and every 2 to 3 mo going forward. Laser treatment and electrolysis are also options, with better results when used in conjunction with COCP.[3,10,16]

Treatment for acne and androgenic alopecia overlap with that for hirsutism. COCP and spironolactone are effective for these conditions. Flutamide is also indicated for androgen related alopecia as is topical finasteride and minoxidil. Refer to dermatology if treatment for hirsutism, acne, and alopecia are refractory to COCP, spironolactone, and topical agents noted earlier.

CHRONIC ANOVULATION

The first line treatment is COCP. Providers should choose the lowest effective estrogen (20–30 mcg of ethinyl estradiol).[16,29] Consider efficacy, metabolic risk profile, and risk assessment for VTE when making selection. Progesterone only therapy, intrauterine device (IUD) and Nexplanon, Depo-provera, or continuous progestin pill should be considered if COCP is not tolerated. These options are good for endometrial protection but have a limited effect on reducing hyperandrogenism.[16,24] Refer to gynecology for IUD and Nexplanon. Last option is cyclic progestin therapy[16,24] Patient is prescribed medroxyprogesterone acetate 5 to 10 mg for 10 to 14 d every 1 to 2 mo, which targets endometrial protection and induces uterine bleeding.[16,29] This does not prevent pregnancy or help with androgenic effects. It is worth mentioning that Metformin can restore ovulation in approximately 30% to 50% of women.[24]

OBESITY

Lifestyle is a major factor that should be emphasized with patients. Weight loss can be challenging in this population, but there are significant benefits to losing weight. A loss of 5% to 10% of weight can restore ovulatory cycles, decrease insulin resistance, lower blood pressure and lipids, and lower risk for OSA and cardiovascular risk.[5,26,29] There is no consensus on which diet is superior in this population. A registered dietician can help prescribe a healthy diet. A healthy diet should be coupled with exercise. 150 to 300 min of moderate intensity or 75 to 150 min of high intensity exercise per week plus resistance training 2 d per week are recommended for prevention of weight gain.[20,29] For weight loss, 250 min of moderate intensity exercise or 150 min of high intensity exercise per week, plus resistance training 2 d per week is recommended.[20,29] Glucagon-like peptide (GLP-1) receptor agonists (liraglutide, semaglutide) and gastric inhibitory polypeptide (GIP) receptor agonist/GLP-1 receptor agonist combo (tirzepatide) are newer anti-obesity medications that have proven to be very effective. These medications help with weight loss and insulin resistance. Insurance coverage can pose a barrier, as most currently do not cover anti-obesity medications. Bariatric surgery is another treatment option.

INSULIN RESISTANCE

Along with weight loss, metformin is a first-line treatment. Metformin is an insulin sensitizer. Used for T2DM, impaired glucose tolerance, hyperandrogenism, ovulation induction, and weight. Stomach upset and diarrhea are possible side effects.[10] An extended-release formulation is available to help decrease the risk of gastric upset. The dosing range is 500 mg daily to 2000 mg daily. Renal function and vitamin B12 levels (with long-term use) should be monitored. GLP-1 receptor agonists and GIP receptor agonists can be used in conjunction with metformin. Inositol, a dietary supplement, may play a role in insulin sensitizing[30] and use is supported by the 2023 International PCOS Guidelines.[16] Currently, there are not enough data to support using it in women with PCOS to help with ovulation, hirsutism, or weight loss.

Dyslipidemia

The primary treatment measures to improve lipid profile are weight loss and lifestyle changes.[26] Statin therapy is an option for those with higher risk of cardiovascular disease. Reliable contraception is required when considering use in women of childbearing age.

Sleep Apnea

Restorative sleep is important for health. Patients with PCOS carry a higher risk of developing OSA.[26] Recommend screening patients when there is a concern and refer to sleep study if warranted. Weight loss and use of continuous positive airway pressure device are the general recommendations for OSA.[26]

NON-ALCOHOLIC FATTY LIVER DISEASE

As with the other conditions noted earlier, weight loss is the main treatment recommendation.[23] Semaglutide has shown positive effects treating non alchoholic steaohepatitis. When appropriate, refer to gastroenterology.

PSYCHOLOGIC SYMPTOMS

PCOS is commonly associated with depression and anxiety.[3,10,29] Psychotherapy and antidepressants are treatment options. Social support groups and organizations for women with PCOS are also available.

VITAMIN D DEFICIENCY/INSUFFICIENCY

Deficiency/insufficiency in vitamin D is common in women with PCOS. Depending on their level, prescription strength vitamin D 2 is available to replete insufficient levels quickly.[31–33] Over-the-counter, vitamin D3 is available to maintain and address deficiencies.[31]

REPRODUCTIVE CONSIDERATIONS
Preconception Risk Factors and Counseling

PCOS is the most common reason for anovulatory infertility.[34] However, those with PCOS should be reassured that pregnancy can be achieved successfully either naturally or with assistance. Optimizing reproductive health early on is imperative by achieving healthy lifestyle, preventing excess weight gain, and mitigating preconception risk factors. Risk factors associated with infertility in those with PCOS include phenotype A, insulin resistance, and obesity/excess weight during pregnancy. Phenotype A is the most severe form of PCOS, which encompasses ovulation dysfunction, elevated androgens, and polycystic ovaries. There is greater resistance to fertility treatments in this phenotype.[35] If insulin resistance is present, there is a higher risk of miscarriage; up to 30% prior to 20 w gestation.[36] This is thought to be due to the inflammatory state of the placenta, it's direct effect on vascular function, and elevated androgen levels. Obesity is the most common co-morbidity seen in pregnancy; it affects more than half of those with fertility issues in PCOS. Those with higher androgens are less likely to ovulate. Other chronic conditions should not be disregarded. Diabetes, hypertension, anxiety, depression, and other mental health conditions should all be optimally managed.

Preconception counseling should include a good nutrition and exercise plan, early identification of diabetes, monitoring blood pressure, taking a higher dose of folic acid to reduce risk of fetal malformation, and optimizing vitamin D. A calcium supplement of 1000 mg daily can reduce blood pressure.[36] Counseling should also include taking acetylsalicylic acid starting at 12 w to reduce occurrence of pre-term and term preeclampsia along with reducing the risk of fetal growth restriction. Women above healthy weight range should achieve 5% to 10% weight loss through 30% energy deficit (500–750 kcal/per day) or 1200 to 1500 kcal/day total intake.[37,38] Weight loss of 10% can often re-establish ovulation. Metformin may restore ovulation in about 50% of those with PCOS (Guan 2020). It also could be considered for use during pregnancy to reduce the risk of preterm birth and limit gestational weight gain.[34] It should be noted that Metformin does not reduce risk for gestational diabetes. Those treated with Metformin must be counseled regarding unclear long-term health effects on offspring and suggestion of increased childhood weight.[34] **Table 5** summarizes preconception counseling for optimizing health and recommendations.

Infertility Treatment Options

Infertility treatment should include both non-pharmacologic and pharmacologic interventions. For those with BMI greater than or equal to 30, weight loss may improve pregnancy outcomes. Other lifestyle interventions include healthy eating and regular exercise. Ovarian induction agents include letrozole (first-line although off-label), clomiphene citrate (CC), Metformin, and GnRH.[34] Before starting infertility treatment, one must have a negative pregnancy test. Explanation of benefits, risks, efficacy, and costs is prudent. The pharmacologic treatment with letrozole for infertility related to PCOS is considered off-label; however, it is now recommended first-line with the available data showing higher live-birth rates with letrozole than clomiphene.[34] CC is an anti-estrogen therapy that blocks estrogen receptors in the hypothalamus and leads to follicular development with negative feedback.[39] Letrozole is an aromatase inhibitor that results in lowering estrogen levels to reduce the risk of multiple follicle development.[39] Metformin can be used to improve clinical pregnancy by reducing insulin resistance and increasing both ovulatory cycles and live birth rates. However, women should know there are more effective ovulation agents.[34] Note that clomiphene citrate + metformin is preferred over one or the other alone to improve live birth

Table 5
Summary of preconception counseling for optimizing health and recommendations[34,36,37]

Preconception Counseling and Health Optimization	Recommendation
Diet and nutritional status	Assess and optimize
Exercise/activity plan	Minimum of 150 min per w at moderate intensity or 75 min per w at vigorous intensity for prevention of weight gain or a min of 250 min per w at moderate intensity or 150 min per w at vigorous intensity for modest weight loss
Weight/weight loss	5%–10% if BMI is over 25 mg/d2
Identifying diabetes early	OGTT either in preconception phase or initial antenatal visit and repeated at 24/28 wk
Monitoring blood pressure	Goal <140/80, if not at goal, then typically treated with labetalol or nifedipine
Prenatal vitamin	In line with routine preconception care
Folate supplementation	0.6 mg/day
Vitamin D3	2000 IU daily reduces insulin resistance, CRP, improves ovulatory function and reproductive potential, decreases risk of low birth weight
Calcium	>1000 mg daily can reduce hypertension
Aspirin 81 mg	Starting at 12 w
Smoking and alcohol status	Assess, counsel, and treat
Sleep	Assess for fatigue, sleep patterns, and sleep apnea
Mental, emotional, and sexual health	Assess, counsel, and treat

rates.[34] There is an association with multiple pregnancies when using CC and monitoring requires use of ultrasound.[39]

Gonadotropins can be considered as second-line therapy alongside CC or in those that are CC resistant. A low-dose step-up approach is followed to reduce the risk of ovarian hyperstimulation syndrome (OHSS) and multiple pregnancies.[39] Cycle monitoring, injection burden, and cost can be factors associated with the choice of gonadotrophin therapy.[34]

Ovarian drilling has a mechanism of action that is not fully understood. It appears that the puncturing of the ovaries in this technique impairs local androgen synthesis, thus reducing androgen levels. This lowers the peripheral conversion to estrogen and decreases the positive feedback on LH secretion. Drilling improves irregular cycles and occurrence of ovulation and pregnancy. It may be considered as second-line therapy with CC resistance.

If first or second-line therapies fail, in vitro fertilization (IVF)/intracytoplasmic sperm injection can be offered. Multiple pregnancies can be reduced if single embryo transfer is used.[34] There is also increased risk of OHSS if IVF is used.[39] In in vitro maturation, OHSS and multiple pregnancies can be avoided, which is particularly appealing in those that need to minimize exposure to estrogen such as women with breast cancer or thrombophilia.[39] However, there is a lower cumulative live birth rate than IVF.[39] **Fig. 1** summarizes reproductive treatment options.

Pregnancy Outcomes (Relative to Polycystic Ovary Syndrome)

Those with PCOS have a 3 to 5-fold increase in risk for adverse pregnancy outcomes when compared with those without PCOS. Therefore, proper monitoring and support

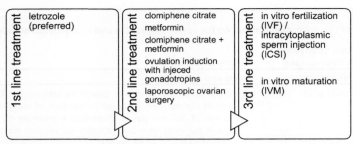

Fig. 1. Summary of reproductive treatment.[34,39]

is needed. The risks include miscarriage, preterm birth, higher gestational weight gain, pregnancy induced hypertension, pre-eclampsia, gestational diabetes (especially with preexisting hyperinsulinemia), and need for caesarean section.[34] The risk of miscarriage is higher if insulin resistance is present, with a loss rate as high as 30%.[36] There is a 2-fold increased risk of preterm birth, especially in those with gestational diabetes.[40–42] Insulin resistance and hyperandrogenism contribute to developing pregnancy induced hypertension.[43] Pregnancy outcomes include those that can both affect the mother and/or the baby. Adverse fetal outcomes include intrauterine growth restriction, small for gestational age, low birth weight, stillbirth, preterm birth as aforementioned, and other anomalies, which can include neural tube defects, congenital heart defects, and neuro-developmental delay.[41,44]

An important piece to consider is that pregnancy history may be a way to predict the future as it relates to health issues in those with PCOS. A review was done of 22 studies, which included 6 million women that showed the aforementioned risks are associated with the development of diabetes within the decade following pregnancy, 3-fold risk of developing hypertension, 2-fold risk of cerebrovascular accident, 40% increased risk of developing heart disease, and 4-fold risk of heart failure. Combined, the risk of pregnancy outcomes discussed here are associated with premature mortality.[28]

SUMMARY

PCOS is a complex disorder that remains under-recognized and under-diagnosed. Failure of providers to recognize, diagnose, and treat PCOS can have adverse health outcomes for this population.[5,9] It is important to keep in mind that PCOS is a long-term condition with increased co-morbidities that can affect both physical health and mental health. Support and care for this population begins with identifying adolescents/women who present with menstrual concerns and features of hyperandrogenism, ruling out other conditions and then creating a collaborative care plan. Treatment, counseling, and preventative care to mitigate health risks in this population are crucial. A multidisciplinary team approach offers the greatest opportunity for addressing care needs, reducing co-morbidity risk, and improving quality-of-life.

CLINICS CARE POINTS

- There are different criteria for diagnosing PCOS, with Rotterdam being the most widely used.
- PCOS is a diagnosis of exclusion as clinical features of PCOS can mirror other conditions. Features of PCOS include menstrual irregularities, hirsutism, acne, and androgenic-related alopecia.

- PCOS is not limited to a reproductive disorder.
- Delays in diagnosis can add to the psychologic symptoms associated with PCOS. Early recognition and diagnosis of PCOS can help decrease risk factors for co-morbidities.
- Hold hormonal contraception for at least 3 mo prior to checking total and free testosterone, LH, and FSH. Use high quality assays for checking testosterone levels.
- Hold biotin supplement prior to checking thyroid function to avoid laboratory assay interference.
- Check vitamin B12 levels with long-term use of metformin.
- Counsel that GLP-1 RA/GIP can help insulin sensitizing and weight loss; however, they are not used during pregnancy.

DISCLOSURE

The authors have nothing to disclosures.

REFERENCES

1. Deswal R, Narwal V, Dang A, et al. The prevalence of polycystic ovary syndrome: a brief systemic review. Reprod Sci 2020;13:261–71.
2. Emanuel RHK, Roberts J, Docherty PD, et al. A review of the hormones involved in the endocrine dysfunctions of polycystic ovary syndrome and their interactions. Front Endocrinol 2022;13:1017468.
3. Sadghi HM, Adeli I, Calina D, et al. Polycystic ovary syndrome: a comprehensive review of pathogenisis, management, and drug repurposing. Int J Mol Sci 2022; 23:583.
4. Barber TM. Why are women with polycystic ovary syndrome obese? Br Med Bull 2022;143:4–14.
5. Witchel SF, Teede HJ, Pena AS. Curtailing PCOS. Pediatr Res 2020;87(1): 353–61.
6. Jabeen A, Yamin V, Amberina AR, et al. Polycystic ovarian syndrome: prevalence, predisposing factors, and awareness among adolescent and young girls of south India. Cureus 2022;14(8):e27943.
7. Sydora BC, Wilke MS, McPherson M, et al. Challenges in diagnosis and health care in polycystic ovary syndrome in Canada: a patient view to improve health care. BMC Wom Health 2023;23:569.
8. Bulsara J, Patel P, Soni A, Acharya S. A review: Brief insight into Polycystic Ovarian syndrome. Endocrinol Metab 2021;3:100085.
9. Sanchez-Garrido MA, Tena-Sempere M. Metabolic dysfunction in polycystic ovary syndrome: Pathogenic role of androgen excess and potential therapeutic strategies. Mol Metab 2020;35:100937.
10. Kamenov Z, Gateva A. Insitols in PCOS. Molecules 2020;25:5566.
11. Islam H, Masud J, Islam YN, Haque FKM. An update on polycystic ovary syndrome: A review of the current state of knowledge in diagnosis, genetic etiology, and emergency treatment options. Women's Heath 2022;18:1–23.
12. Tremblay-Davis AC, Holley SL, Downes LA. Diagnosis and treatment of polycystic ovary syndrome in primary care. J Nurse Pract 2021;17(10):1226–9.
13. Barbieri R.L., Simplify your approach to the diagnosis and treatment of PCOS. OBG Management, vol. 34, no. 12, 2022, pp. 9+. Gale Academic OneFile Select,

Available at: link.gale.com/apps/doc/A732713537/EAIM?u=duke_perkins&-sid=bookmark-EAIM&xid=54caf97f. (Accessed 6 March 2024).

14. Dapas M., Dunaif A., Deconstructing a syndrome: Genomic Insights Into PCOS Causal Mechanisms and Classification. Endocrine Reviews, 43, no. 6, 2022, pp. 927+. Gale Academic OneFile, link.gale.com/apps/doc/A767645255/AONE?u=duke_perkins&sid=summon&xid=8673af21.

15. Kakkad V, Reddy NS, Nihlani H, Gundewar T. Age-related diagnostic threshold of anti-Müllerian hormone for polycystic ovarian syndrome. Int J Gynecol Obstet 2021;153:443–8.

16. Vine D, Ghosh M, Wang T, Bakal J. Increased prevalence of adverse health outcomes across the lifespan in those affected by polycystic ovary syndrome: a canadian population cohort. CJC 2024;314–26.

17. Shabaz M, Almatoog H, Foucambert P, et al. A systematic review of the risk of non-alcoholic fatty liver disease in women with polycystic ovary syndrome. Cureus 2022;14(10):e29928.

18. Witchel SF, Oberfield SE, Peña A. Polycystic ovary syndrome: pathophysiology, presentation, and treatment with emphasis on adolescent girls. J Endocr Soc 2019;3(8):1545–73.

19. Teede HJ, Tay CT, Laven JJE, et al. International Recommendation from 2023 International evidenced-based guideline for the assessment and management of polycystic ovary syndrome. Eur J Endocrinol 2023;189(2):G43–64.

20. Osibogun O, Ogunmoroti O, Michos ED. Polycystic ovary syndrome and cardiometabolic risk: opportunities for cardiovascular disease prevention. Trends Cardiovasc Med 2020;30(7):399–404.

21. Ollila MM, Arffman RK, Korhonen E, et al. Women with PCOS have an increased risk for cardiovascular disease regardless of diagnostic criteria-a prospective population-based cohort study. Eur J Endocrinol 2023;189(1):96–105.

22. Mitra S, Saharia GK, Jena SK. Cardio-metabolic risk in Rotterdam clinical phenotypes of PCOS. Ann Endocrinol (Paris) 2024;85(1):44–7.

23. Vural F, Vural B, Kardaş E, et al. The diagnostic performance of antimullerian hormone for polycystic ovarian syndrome and polycystic ovarian morphology. Arch Gynecol Obstet 2023;307:1083–90.

24. Recommendations from the 2023 International Evidenced-based guideline for the assessment and management of polycystic ovary syndrome (2023), Available at: https://www.asrm.org/practice-guidance/practice-committee-documents/recommendations-from-the-2023-international-evidence-based-guideline-for-the-assessment-and-management-of-polycystic-ovary-syndrome/. (Accessed 6 March 2024).

25. Carmina E. Need to introduce the finding of obesity or normal body weight in the current diagnostic criteria and in the classification of PCOS. Diagnostics 2022; 12(10):2555.

26. Pea J, Bryan J, Wan C, et al. Ultrasonographic criteria in the diagnosis of polycystic ovary syndrome: a systematic review and diagnostic meta-analysis. Hum Reprod Update 2024;30(1):109–30.

27. Farland LV, Stern JE, Liu CL, et al. Polycystic ovary syndrome and risk of adverse pregnancy outcomes: a registry linkage study from Massachusetts. Hum Reprod 2022;37(11):2690–9.

28. Guan Y, Wang D, Bu H. The Effect of Metformin on Polycystic Ovary Syndrome in Overweight Women: a Systematic Review and Meta-Analysis of Randomized Controlled Trials. Int J Endocrinol 2020;2020:5150684.

29. Akre S, Sharma K, Chakole S, Wanjari MB. Recent advances in the management of polycystic ovary syndrome: a review article. Cureus 2022;14(8):e27689.
30. Martin KA, Anderson RR, Chang RJ, et al. Evaluation and treatment of hirsutism in premenopausal women: an endocrine society clinical practice guideline. J Clin Endocrinol Metab 2018;103(4):1233–57.
31. Minocha N. Polycystic ovarian disease or polycystic ovarian syndrome: how to identify and manage-a review. Archives of Pharmacy Practice 2020;11(2–2020): 102–6.
32. Mohan A, Haider R, Fakhor H, et al. Vitamin D and polycystic ovary syndrome (PCOS): a review. Ann Med Surg (Lond) 2023;85(7):3506–11.
33. Cowan S, Lim S, Alycia C, et al. Lifestyle management in polycystic ovary syndrome–beyond diet and physical activity. BMC Endocr Disord 2023;23(1):14.
34. Teede HJ, Misso ML, Costello MF, et al. Recommendations from the international evidence-based guideline for the assessment and management of polycystic ovary syndrome. Hum Reprod 2018;33(9):1602–18.
35. Ajmal N, Khan SZ, Shaikh R. Polycystic ovary syndrome (PCOS) and genetic predisposition: a review article. Eur J Obstet Gynecol Reprod Biol X 2019;3:100060.
36. Mayrhofer D, Hager M, Walch K, et al. The prevalence and impact of polycystic ovary syndrome in recurrent miscarriage: a retrospective cohort study and meta-analysis. J Clin Med 2020;9(9):2700.
37. Joham A, Norman R, Stener-Victorin E, et al. Polycystic ovary syndrome. Lancet Diabetes Endocrinol 2022;10(9):668–80.
38. Collée J, Mawet M, Tebache L, et al. Polycystic ovarian syndrome and infertility: overview and insights of the putative treatments. Gynecol Endocrinol 2021; 37(10):869–74.
39. Chen X, Gissler M, Lavebratt C. Association of maternal polycystic ovary syndrome and diabetes with preterm birth and offspring birth size: a population-based cohort study. Hum Reprod 2022;37(6):1311–23.
40. Mills G, Badeghiesh A, Suarthana E, et al. Polycystic ovary syndrome as an independent risk factor for gestational diabetes and hypertensive disorders of pregnancy: a population-based study on 9.1 million pregnancies. Hum Reprod 2020; 35(7):1666–74.
41. Mills G, Badeghiesh A, Suarthana E, et al. Associations between polycystic ovary syndrome and adverse obstetric and neonatal outcomes: a population study of 9.1 million births. Hum Reprod 2020;35(8):1914–21.
42. Wekker V, van Dammen L, Koning A, et al. Long-term cardiometabolic disease risk in women with PCOS: a systematic review and meta-analysis. Hum Reprod Update 2020;26(6):942–60.
43. Subramanian A, Lee SI, Phillips K, et al. Polycystic ovary syndrome and risk of adverse obstetric outcomes: a retrospective population-based matched cohort study in England. BMC Med 2022;20(1):298.
44. Hillman SC, Bryce C, Caleyachetty R, Dale J. Women's experiences of diagnosis and management of polycystic ovary syndrome: a mixed-methods study in general practice. Br J Gen Pract 2020;70(694):e322–9.

Psychometric Scales of the Strong Black Woman Construct Evaluating Stress-Related Health Disparities among African American Women

A Scoping Review

Amnazo Muhirwa, PhD, MSN, FNP-C, BSN, RN[a,*],
Cheryl Giscombe, PhD, RN, PMHNP-BC[b,c],
Devon Noonan, PhD, MPH, FNP-BC, CARN, FIAAN[d], Susan Silva, PhD[e],
Bradi Granger, PhD, RN[f]

KEYWORDS

- Strong Black woman • Superwoman schema • African American women
- Gendered racism • Stress measurement • Health disparities
- Psychometric evaluation • Women's health intervention

KEY POINTS

- This scoping review explores the use of psychometric measures to assess the strong Black woman and superwoman constructs among African American women.
- It identifies and evaluates various scales utilized in existing literature, highlighting their strengths, limitations, and clinical implications for women's health.
- The review emphasizes the importance of incorporating culturally relevant measures of stress into clinical practice to better understand and address the unique stressors experienced by Black women.

Continued

---

[a] Program on Integrative Medicine, Department of Physical Medicine & Rehabilitation, University of North Carolina School of Medicine, Carrington Hall, CB#7460, Chapel Hill, NC 27599-7460, USA; [b] Office of Academic Affairs, UNC Chapel Hill School of Nursing, Carrington Hall, CB#7460, Chapel Hill, NC 27599-7460, USA; [c] Department of Social Medicine, School of Medicine, Carrington Hall, CB#7460, Chapel Hill, NC 27599-7460, USA; [d] Duke National Clinician Scholars Program, Duke School of Nursing, Duke Cancer Institute, Cancer Control and Population Sciences, 307 Trent Drive, Durham, NC 27710, USA; [e] Duke University School of Nursing, 307 Trent Drive, Durham, NC 27710, USA; [f] Heart Center Nursing Research Program Duke University Health System, Duke-Margolis Center for Health Policy, 307 Trent Drive, Durham, NC 27710, USA
* Corresponding author. Carrington Hall, CB#7460, Chapel Hill, NC 27599-7460.
E-mail address: Amnazo_muhirwa@med.unc.edu

Nurs Clin N Am 59 (2024) 577–592
https://doi.org/10.1016/j.cnur.2024.07.006
0029-6465/24/© 2024 Elsevier Inc. All rights are reserved, including those for text and data mining, AI training, and similar technologies.

Continued

- By recognizing and validating the experiences of Black women, health care providers can tailor interventions to promote holistic well-being and mitigate the adverse effects of stress on health outcomes.
- Overall, the article underscores the need for further research and clinical application of these measures to improve health outcomes and health care access for Black women.

INTRODUCTION

African American women face significantly higher rates of stress-related chronic health conditions compared to their White counterparts.[1-6] They are more prone to obesity, diabetes, cardiovascular diseases, and other stress-related ailments, which are exacerbated by repeated exposure to stressors.[2,5,7] Research over the past 2 decades has underscored the links between psychological stress and adverse health outcomes in African American women,[8,9] elucidating the intricate relationships among stress, health behaviors, and psychophysiological processes.[10,11] Notably, stress in African American women, including race-related and gender-related stress, has been associated with inadequate physical activity and stress-related eating behaviors, contributing to increased risk for obesity and chronic illness.[12,13]

The concepts of the strong Black woman (SBW) and superwoman are often used interchangeably. The SBW embodies an ideal of Black womanhood, symbolizing strength and resilience while shouldering multiple roles within her family and community.[14,15] This archetype is characterized by silent suffering and the pressure to fulfill societal expectations without expressing vulnerability or seeking help.[16] Many African American women cope with their burdens in silence or through inefficient coping mechanisms to maintain their perceived strength within their communities.[14,17,18] Multiple role stress further compounds this burden, as women juggle various identities and responsibilities,[13] contributing to cumulative stress.

Scholars argue that the superwoman/SBW role reflects a stance of resilience and self-efficacy adopted to navigate life's adversities, underscoring its importance in understanding the complex dynamics of African American women's health.[4,14,19,20] However, despite burgeoning research, there remains a need for more studies to elucidate the mechanisms linking stress to health outcomes in African American women, necessitating culturally and contextually relevant measures of stress. Therefore, this scoping review aims to identify studies employing psychometric measures of the "SBW" or "superwoman" construct to assess stress-related disparities among African American women.

METHODS
Design

A scoping review of the literature was utilized, guided by the methodological framework of Arksey and O'Malley,[10] to identify relevant gaps in the literature and the current research standing of the topic. The population identified studies involving adult women who identify as Black and/or African American, aged 18 years and over, and psychometrically measured the SBW/superwoman construct. Preferred Reporting Items for Systematic Reviews and Meta-Analyses reporting guidelines for scoping reviews were followed.[21] Following the PRISAM guidelines (Moher, Liberati, Tetzlaff, & Altman,

2009),[21] a search was conducted in the electronic bibliographic databases PsycINFO, PubMed, Ovid MEDLINE, Embase, and Cumulative Index to Nursing Allied Health Literature (CINAHL) to identity relevant articles. The search terms comprised the key words in a variety of combinations: "Strong black woman, superwoman, stereotypical role, gender role, gendered racism, psychological, stress, stressors." The search was limited to only peer-reviewed articles, articles in English language, published between 2000 and 2020, and measuring the SBW/superwoman construct. The complete, reproducible search strategy for all databases is available in Appendix 1.

Two phases were used to complete the scoping review. The first phase included title and abstract screening and the second phase included a full-text screening of the selected articles. After reviewing the articles' titles and abstracts, 119 articles were available for full-text review. After the full-text screening was conducted, it was determined that 13 articles met all inclusion criteria. From each study meeting the inclusion criteria, information on author, year, and journal of publication, country in which study was conducted, the measure of SBW/superwoman used in the study and psychometric properties of the measure (if documented) was extracted and charted into Microsoft Office Excel. For psychometric data, we extracted Cronbach's alpha, intra-class coefficient of correlation, or any other correlation coefficient, if reported, when documenting the reliability of a given measure. Where a study explored the validity of a given measure of SBW/superwoman, we documented the type of validity examined such as construct, content, criterion, concurrent, divergent, or convergent validity, alongside supporting statistics.

Data Extraction

We utilized Covidence to screen articles by title and abstract. Two researchers independently conducted the screening process and resolved any discrepancies through discussion. Full-text articles of the selected studies were then screened, and all included articles were used in the final analysis of the scoping review. Given the nature of the review, critical appraisal of study quality was not performed.[22] Data extraction included information on author(s), publication year, study location, study population characteristics, aims, methodology, outcome measures, and key results. **Table 1** summarizes the inclusion and exclusion criteria used: SBW/superwoman scales were included. Scales examining partial characteristics of the SBW/superwoman construct were also included.

Table 1
Inclusion and exclusion criteria for scoping review

Inclusion Criteria	Exclusion Criteria
English-language studies published in a peer-reviewed journal between January 01, 2000 and December 31, 2020.	Studies examining only psychometric properties of strong Black woman/superwoman scales, including validation, development, and assessment.
Quantitatively (objectively) measuring strong Black woman/superwoman construct.	Qualitative assessment of strong Black woman/superwoman.
Participants are women identifying as Black and/or African American woman aged 18 years and older.	Outside of the United States.
Association to some stress-related health outcome.	

Data Analysis

To analyze the literature, 2 researchers collaborated to identify the main topics and themes across the included studies. This involved charting key information obtained from the primary research reports, such as the intended constructs measured by the scales. Consistency in construct definitions was maintained through rigorous consensus among all authors.

RESULTS
Study Selection

A total of 789 articles were initially included in the search for relevant scales (**Fig. 1**). Following screening and full-text review, 13 studies met the inclusion criteria and were included in the final analysis.

Scales Used to Operationalize Strong Black Woman/Superwoman

Table 2 summarizes the key findings across studies. Among the 13 studies, 7 utilized the Stereotypic Roles for Black Women Scale (SRBWS),[33] while 2 study used the Giscombe Superwoman Schema Questionnaire (G-SWS-Q),[14] and 3 used the Gendered

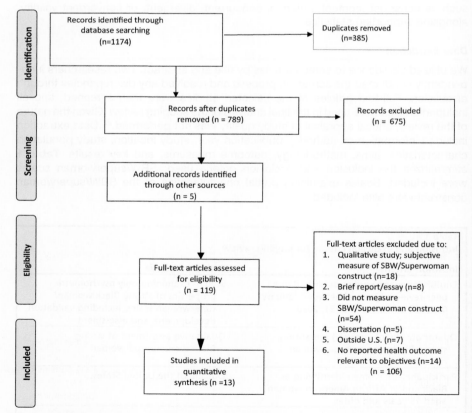

Fig. 1. Preferred reporting items for systematic reviews and meta-analyses flow diagram of scoping review.

Table 2
Key findings across studies

Author(s), Year	Scale	# Of Items	Psychometric Properties	Study Location and Population	Aims/Purpose
Knighton et al,[23] 2020	Modified Stereotypic Roles for Black Women Scale (strength/suppress emotions): 4 point Likert scale ranging from 1 = strongly agree to 4 = strongly disagree.	10	α = .88	Historically Black colleges and universities, colleges and universities in a southern state (United States) 243 African American women 19–72 years old (M = 39.49, SD = 12.59)	Investigating obligation to show strength/suppress emotion as a potential mediator between racial microaggressions and psychological distress among middle-class African American women.
Abrams, et al,[26] 2018	Stereotypic Roles of Black Women Scale (superwoman subscale): 5 point point Likert scale ranging from 1 (strongly disagree) to 5.	11	α = .78	United States 194 African American women 18–82 years old (M = 37.53, SD = 19.88)	Investigated whether self-silencing mediates the relation between perceived strength obligations and depression.
Allen et al,[2] 2019	The Giscombe Superwoman Schema Questionnaire (G-SWS-Q) 4 point Likert scale ranging from 0 = "This is not true for me" to 3 = "This is true for me all the time"	35	α = .76–.89	San Francisco Bay area 207 African American women 30–50 years old (M = 41.72)	Examined whether the superwoman schema (SWS) modifies the association between racial discrimination and allostatic load

(continued on next page)

Table 2
(continued)

Author(s), Year	Scale	# Of Items	Psychometric Properties	Study Location and Population	Aims/Purpose
Giscombe et al,[25] 2019	The Giscombe Superwoman Schema Questionnaire (G-SWS-Q)	35	Obligation to present an image of strength: Cronbach's alpha appraisal α = .70 Obligation to suppress emotions: Cronbach's alpha appraisal α = .85 Resistance to being vulnerable: Cronbach's alpha appraisal α = .86 Intense motivation to succeed: Cronbach's alpha appraisal α = .72 Obligation to help others: Cronbach's alpha appraisal α = .87	hair salons, civic and church organizations, and via listserv groups 130 African American women 18–75 years old (M = 41.19, SD = 14.74)	Described the psychometric evaluation of the G-SWS-Q, based on the 5 dimensions of the Superwoman Schema Conceptual Framework.
Dale et al,[28] 2019	*GRMS—Black women (GRMS—BW):* 5 point Likert scale ranging from 0 = never, to 5 = once a week or more 5 point Likert scale ranging from 0 = never happened to 5 = extremely stressful).	32	appraisal α = 0.93 and frequency α = 0.92)	Large urban city in the Southeastern United States 100 African American M = 49.25 (SD = 10.89, 22–67)	Aimed to bridge the gap in the literature by providing insight into the relationships among racial discrimination, HIV-related discrimination, and GRMS and barriers to HIV-related care among Black Women Living with HIV

| Dale & Safren,[27] 2019 | Gendered Racial Microaggressions Scale for Black Women 5 point Likert scale ranging from 0 = never, to 5 = once a week or more 5 point Likert scale ranging from 0 = never happened to 5 = extremely stressful). | 26 | Cronbach's alpha appraisal α = .95 Frequency α = .92 | Large urban metropolitan area in the Southeastern United States 100 BWLWH M = 49 (range = 22–67) | Investigated the associations among Gendered Racial Microaggresions, race-related and HIV-related discrimination, and trauma symptoms among BWLWH and explored whether gendered racial microaggressions contributed uniquely to trauma symptoms above the contribution of race-related and HIV-related discrimination. |
| Jerald et al,[24] 2017 | Modern Jezebel Scale adapted from the Stereotypic Roles of Black Women Scale To assess women's awareness of the Jezebel and Sapphire stereotypes 5 point Likert scale ranging from 1 (strongly disagree) to 5. Modified version of Strong Black Woman Scale–Endorsement: To assess women's awareness of the SBW ideology 5 point Likert scale ranging from 1 (strongly disagree) to 5. | 12 (Jezebel) 12 (Sapphire) 9 (Strong Black Woman Scale–Endorsement) | Jezebel subscale α = .95 Sapphire subscale α = .97 Modified SBW Scale subscale α = .90 | Two college campuses in the United States 609 African American Woman M = 22.13 (SD = 5.32). | Examined how Black women's metastereotype awareness, that is, awareness that others hold stereotypes of their group, influences mental health, self-care, and substance use for coping. Also examined the moderating role of racial identity in these associations |

(continued on next page)

Table 2
(continued)

Author(s), Year	Scale	# Of Items	Psychometric Properties	Study Location and Population	Aims/Purpose
Lewis et al,[29] 2017	*Gendered racial microaggressions*: 6 point Likert-type response ranging from 0 (never) to 5 (once a week or more). *Gendered racial identity centrality*: modified version of the 10 item Multidimensional Inventory of Black Identity Centrality subscale to measure the intersection of racial and gender identity centrality. 7 point Likert-type scale ranging from 1 (strongly disagree) to 7 (strongly agree).	26 (gendered microaggression); 10 (gendered racial centrality)	Cronbach's alpha reliability estimate α = .92 (gendered microaggression) Cronbach's alpha coefficient α = .80 (gendered racial centrality)	Online US Survey—(54%) Southeast, 18% Midwest, 17% Northeast, and 10% West Coast 231 Black women 37 y (SD = 12.38)	The purpose of this study was to apply an intersectionality framework to explore the influence of gendered racism (ie, intersection of racism and sexism) on health outcomes
Watson & Hunter,[30] 2015	SBW race-gender schema: 5 point Likert-type scale ranging from 1 (strongly disagree) to 5 (strongly agree).	11 item Superwoman subscale and 5 item Mammy subscale were combined to measure the SBW race-gender schema	Cronbach's alpha reliability α = .77	Local Midwest university and rural community for the study 95 African American women 18 and 65 y (M = 20.91, SD = 7.27)	investigated whether African American women's endorsement of the SBW race-gender schema predicted increased symptoms of anxiety and depression and whether attitudes toward professional psychological help-seeking intensified psychological distress

Study	Scale	Items	Reliability	Sample/Setting	Purpose
Brown et al,[31] 2013	*Modern Jezebel stereotype:* 5 point Likert scale ranging from strongly disagree (1) to strongly agree (5).	7	Cronbach's alpha $\alpha = 0.82$. Test-retest correlation (r ¼ 0.45, p, 0.001) at 6 months	Online Survey—Midwest region of the United States. 249 African American women. 18–78 y ($M = 38.98$, $SD = 13.64$)	examined generational differences in the endorsement of modern depictions of the Jezebel, as well as the relationship between racial-ethnic esteem and endorsement of this sexualized image.
Donovan & West,[32] 2015	*Stereotypic Roles for Black Women Scale (SRBWS)* 5 point Likert-type scale ranging from 1 = strongly disagree to 5 = strongly agree.	34	Superwoman ($\alpha = .67$), Jezebel ($\alpha = .72$), Sapphire ($\alpha = .70$), Mammy ($\alpha = .53$)	New England University. 92 African American women. 18–47 ($M = 23.32$, $SD = 6.02$)	Examine factors that may be related to African American trauma survivors' binge eating and to identify mechanisms of the associations among trauma, SBW ideology, and binge eating.
Harrington et al,[20] 2010	*Stereotypic Roles for Black Women Scale* (5 point scale (strongly disagree to strongly agree)	11 (Superwoman); 5 (Mammy)	NR	United States: midsized urban hospital internal medicine clinic (27.7%), undergraduate courses at a Midwestern university (52.0%), faculty/staff mailings (14.1%), and word of mouth (6.2%). 179 African American female trauma survivors $M = 29.6$ y, $SD = 12.8$	The goals of this study were to examine factors that may be related to African American trauma survivors' binge eating and to identify mechanisms of the associations among trauma, SBW ideology, and binge eating.

Racial Macroaggressions Scale (GRMS) for Black women.[34] The SRBWS was the most frequently utilized scale.

Stereotypical Roles for Black Women Scale

The SRBWS[33] consists of 34 items assessing endorsement of common stereotypes about African American women across 4 subscales. Not all components of the SRBWS were used consistently across studies.

The Giscombe Superwoman Schema Questionnaire

The G-SWS-Q[14] comprises 35 items grouped into 5 subscales, each representing different dimensions of the superwoman schema. This scale was developed from diverse samples of African American women.

The Gendered Racial Macroaggressions Scale for Black Women

The GRMS[34] assesses gendered racial microaggressions experienced by Black women and consists of 4 subscales. This scale has demonstrated good validity and reliability across multiple studies.

DISCUSSION

The identified scales offer valuable insights into the unique stressors and coping mechanisms experienced by Black women, particularly within the context of the SBW and superwoman constructs. Psychological stress, often stemming from gender-related and race-related factors, has been consistently linked to adverse health outcomes among this population. By utilizing these scales, health care providers can gain a deeper understanding of the multifaceted experiences of Black women and tailor interventions to address their specific needs.

One of the key findings of this scoping review is the variation in scale length and structure. While longer scales may capture a more comprehensive range of experiences, they also run the risk of respondent fatigue and dropout. Conversely, shorter scales may be more accessible and engaging for respondents but may not fully capture the complexity of the constructs being measured. Therefore, it is essential for researchers and clinicians to strike a balance between comprehensiveness and respondent engagement when selecting or developing scales for clinical use.

Furthermore, the predominance of Likert-type scales among the identified measures suggests a preference for assessing subjective experiences and attitudes. While Likert scales offer a convenient way to quantify responses, they may not fully capture the nuances of individual experiences. Future research could explore the use of mixed-method approaches to provide a more comprehensive understanding of the SBW and superwoman constructs, incorporating qualitative data to capture the lived experiences of Black women.

In terms of clinical implications, the findings of this scoping review underscore the importance of incorporating culturally relevant measures of stress into clinical assessments and interventions for Black women. By recognizing and addressing the unique stressors faced by this population, health care providers can improve health outcomes and promote holistic well-being. Additionally, integrating these measures into clinical practice can help identify individuals at risk and tailor interventions to promote healthier behaviors and mitigate the adverse effects of stress on health outcomes.

In conclusion, the scales identified in this scoping review offer valuable tools for clinicians and researchers working to address the contemporary issues in women's health, particularly among Black women. By acknowledging and validating the experiences of Black women, health care providers can create a more inclusive and supportive health care environment that promotes the well-being of all women. Through continued research and clinical application, we can strive toward equitable health care access and outcomes for all women, regardless of race or ethnicity.

LIMITATIONS

Limitations of this review include potential publication bias and the exclusion of scales not using specific terminology. Additionally, the quality of the scales reviewed was not assessed, which may affect the reliability of the findings.

CLINICS CARE POINTS

- The identified scales offer valuable insights into the unique stressors and coping mechanisms experienced by Black women.
- Understanding the interplay between these constructs and health outcomes is crucial for developing effective clinical interventions tailored to the specific needs of Black women.
- Health care providers can utilize these insights to recognize and address silent suffering and multiple role stress experienced by Black women, creating a safe space for them to seek help.
- Integrating culturally relevant measures of stress into clinical practice can help identify individuals at risk and tailor interventions to promote healthier behaviors and mitigate the adverse effects of stress on health outcomes.
- Incorporating measures such as the SBW and superwoman constructs into clinical assessments and interventions can improve health outcomes and promote holistic well-being among Black women.

DISCLOSURES

The authors have nothing to disclose.

REFERENCES

1. Agyemang P, Powell-Wiley TM. Obesity and black women: Special Consider-ations Related to Genesis and therapeutic approaches. Current Cardiovascular Risk Reports 2013;7(5):378–86.
2. Allen AM, Wang Y, Chae DH, et al. Racial discrimination, the superwoman schema, and allostatic load: Exploring an integrative stress-coping model among African American women. Ann N Y Acad Sci 2019;1457(1):104–27.
3. Arksey H, O'Malley L. Scoping studies: Towards a methodological framework. Int J Soc Res Methodol 2005;8(1):19–32.
4. Beauboeuf-Lafontant T. Keeping up appearances, getting fed Up: The embodi-ment of strength among african american women. Meridians Fem race, transna-tionalism 2005;5(2):104–23.
5. Benjamin EJ, Virani SS, Callaway CW, et al. Heart isease and stroke statistics—2018 update: A report from the american heart association. Circulation 2018;137(12).
6. Smilowitz NR, Maduro GA, Lobach IV, et al. Adverse trends in ischemic heart dis-ease mortality among young new yorkers, particularly young black women. PLoS One 2016;11(2):e0149015.
7. Geronimus AT, Hicken MT, Pearson JA, et al. Do US black women experience stress-related accelerated biological aging? Hum Nat 2010;21(1):19–38.

8. Berger M, Sarnyai Z. "More than skin deep": Stress neurobiology and mental health consequences of racial discrimination. Stress 2015;18(1):1–10.

9. Williams DR. Stress and the mental health of populations of color: Advancing our understanding of race-related stressors. J Health Soc Behav 2018;59(4):466–85.

10. Park CL, Iacocca MO. A stress and coping perspective on health behaviors: Theoretical and methodological considerations. Hist Philos Logic 2014;27:123–37.

11. Suls J, Green PA, Boyd CM. Multimorbidity: Implications and directions for health psychology and behavioral medicine. Health Psychol 2019;38(9):772–82.

12. Hammadah M, Sullivan S, Pearce B, et al. Inflammatory response to mental stress and mental stress induced myocardial ischemia. Brain Behav Immun 2018;68:90–7.

13. Sumner JA, Chen Q, Roberts AL, et al. Posttraumatic stress disorder onset and inflammatory and endothelial function biomarkers in women. Brain Behav Immun 2018;69:203–9.

14. Woods-Giscombé CL. Superwoman Schema: African American Women's Views on Stress, Strength, and Health. Qual Health Res 2010;20(5):668–83.

15. Woods-Giscombé CL, Black AR. Mind-body interventions to reduce risk for health disparities related to stress and strength among african american women: The potential of mindfulness-based stress reduction, loving-kindness, and the NTU Therapeutic Framework. Compl Health Pract Rev 2010;15(3):115–31.

16. Huddleston-Mattai B. The black female academician and the 'superwoman syndrome'. Race, Gender & Class 1995;3(1):49–64. Available at: http://www.jstor.org/stable/41675346.

17. Jefferies K. The strong black woman: Insights and implications for nursing. J Am Psychiatr Nurses Assoc 2022;28(4):332–8.

18. Woods-Giscombe Cheryl, Nicolle Robinson M, Carthon D, et al. Superwoman Schema, Stigma, Spirituality, and Culturally Sensitive Providers: Factors influencing african american women's use of mental health services. J Best Pract Health Prof Divers 2016;9(1):1124–44. Available at: https://www.jstor.org/stable/26554242.

19. Edge D, Rogers A. Dealing with it: Black caribbean women's response to adversity and psychological distress associated with pregnancy, childbirth, and early motherhood. Soc Sci Med 2005;61(1):15–25.

20. Harrington EF, Crowther JH, Shipherd JC. Trauma, binge eating, and the "strong Black woman.". J Consult Clin Psychol 2010;78(4):469–79.

21. Moher D, Liberati A, Tetzlaff J, et al, PRISMA Group. Preferred reporting items for systematic reviews and meta-analyses: the PRISMA statement. PLoS Med 2009; 6(7):e1000097.

22. Pham MT, Rajić A, Greig JD, et al. A scoping review of scoping reviews: Advancing the approach and enhancing the consistency. Res Synth Methods 2014;5(4):371–85.

23. Knighton JS, Dogan J, Hargons C, et al. Superwoman Schema: a context for understanding psychological distress among middle-class African American women who perceive racial microaggressions. Ethn Health 2020;27(4):946–62.

24. Jerald MC, Cole ER, Ward LM, et al. Controlling images: How awareness of group stereotypes affects Black women's well-being. J Counsel Psychol 2017;64(5):487–99.

25. Woods-Giscombe CL, Allen AM, Black AR, et al. The Giscombe Superwoman Schema Questionnaire: Psychometric Properties and Associations with Mental Health and Health Behaviors in African American Women. Issues Ment Health Nurs 2019;40(8):672–81.

26. Abrams JA, Hill A, Maxwell M. Underneath the Mask of the Strong Black Woman Schema: Disentangling Influences of Strength and Self-Silencing on Depressive Symptoms among U.S. Black Women. Sex Roles 2019;80(9–10):517–26.
27. Dale SK, Safren SA. Gendered racial microaggressions predict posttraumatic stress disorder symptoms and cognitions among Black women living with HIV. Psychol Trauma Theory Res Pract Policy 2019;11(7):685–94.
28. Dale SK, Dean T, Sharma R, et al. Microaggressions and discrimination relate to barriers to care among black women living with HIV. AIDS Patient Care STDS 2019;33(4):175–83.
29. Lewis JA, Williams MG, Peppers EJ, et al. Applying intersectionality to explore the relations between gendered racism and health among Black women. J Counsel Psychol 2017;64(5):475–86.
30. Watson NN, Hunter CD. Anxiety and depression among African American women: The costs of strength and negative attitudes toward psychological help-seeking. Cult Divers Ethnic Minor Psychol 2015;21(4):604–12.
31. Brown DL, White-Johnson RL, Griffin-Fennell FD. Breaking the chains: examining the endorsement of modern Jezebel images and racial-ethnic esteem among African American women. Cult Health Sex 2013;15(5/6):525–39.
32. Donovan RA, West LM. Stress and Mental Health: Moderating Role of the Strong Black Woman Stereotype. J Black Psychol 2015;41(4):384–96.
33. Thomas AJ, Witherspoon KM, Speight SL. Toward the development of the stereotypic roles for black Women scale. J Black Psychol 2004;30(3):426–42.
34. Lewis Jioni, Neville Helen. Construction and initial validation of the gendered racial microaggressions scale for black women. J Counsel Psychol 2015;62:289–302.

APPENDIX 1: SEARCH STRATEGY REPORT

Topic: Superwoman and African American Women.
 Date: September 9, 2020.
 Note: limited to exclude books/book chapters, magazines, and dissertations.
 Total # of References: 1174.
 # of Duplicates Removed: 385.
 Total # of References to Screen: 789.

Database: MEDLINE (via Ovid)

Set #	(20,658,804 OR 25844565 OR 20154298 OR 30760942 OR 31403707 OR 32176969 OR 31086431 OR 31081707 OR 30507209).ui.	Results 9
1 Black/African American	exp African Americans/	54,277
2	("African American" or "African American" or "African Americans" or "African Americans" or Black or Blacks).ti,ab,kw.	187,089
3	1 OR 2	200,968
4 women	exp female/or exp women/or exp mothers/	8,758,463
5	(female or females or women or women or woman or women's or women or wife or wives or mother or mothers or daughter or daughters).ti,ab,kw.	2,177,374
6	4 OR 5	9,170,003

(continued on next page)

	(20,658,804 OR 25844565 OR 20154298 OR 30760942 OR 31403707 OR 32176969 OR 31086431 OR 31081707 OR	**Results**
Set #	**30507209).ui.**	**9**
7 measures	exp "Surveys and Questionnaires"/	1,040,537
8 measures	(Schema or schemas or scale or scales or framework or frameworks or questionnaire or questionnaires or inventory or inventories or survey or surveys or tool or tools or measure or measures).ti,ab,kw.	3,457,293
9 measures	7 OR 8	3,933,918
10 measures	("strong black woman" or "strong black" or superwoman or "super woman" or "stereotypical role" or "stereotypical roles" or "gender role" or "gender roles" or "gendered racism" or "gendered racial" or sociocultural).ti,ab,kw.	11,812
11 measures	9 AND 10	5261
12 Measures/scales	("superwoman schema" or "strong black woman schema" or "Stereotypic Roles for Black Women Scale" or SRBWS or SBW or "Strong Black Women race gender schema" or "African American Women s Shifting Scale" or AAWSS or "Strong Black Woman Cultural Construct Scale" or SBWCCS or "Gendered Racial Macroaggressions Scale" or GRMS or "Belgrave Gender Role Inventory" or BGRI or "gender role beliefs" or "gender role belief").ti,ab,kw.	302
13 measures	**11 OR 12**	1297
14	**3 AND 6 AND 13**	285

Database: Embase (via Elsevier)

Set #		Results
1	'african american'/de OR 'african american' OR 'african american':ti,ab OR 'african americans':ti,ab OR black:ti,ab OR blacks:ti,ab	275,815
2	'female'/de OR female:ti,ab OR 'females'/de OR females:ti,ab OR 'womans':ti,ab OR 'women'/de OR 'women':ti,ab OR 'woman'/de OR 'woman':ti,ab OR 'women s:ti,ab' OR 'womens':ti,ab OR 'wife'/de OR wife:ti,ab OR wives:ti,ab OR 'mother'/de OR mother:ti,ab OR 'mothers'/de OR 'daughter'/de OR daughter:ti,ab OR 'daughters'/de OR daughters:ti,ab	10,138,270
3	'questionnaire'/de OR Schema:ti,ab or schemas:ti,ab or scale:ti,ab or scales:ti,ab or framework:ti,ab or frameworks:ti,ab or Questionnaire:ti,ab or Questionnaires:ti,ab or inventory:ti,ab or inventories:ti,ab or survey:ti,ab or surveys:ti,ab or tool:ti,ab or tools:ti,ab or measure:ti,ab or measures:ti,ab	4,689,629
4	"strong black woman":ti,ab or "strong black":ti,ab or superwoman:ti,ab or "super woman":ti,ab or "stereotypical role":ti,ab or "stereotypical roles":ti,ab or "gender role":ti,ab or "gender roles":ti,ab or "gendered racism":ti,ab or "gendered racial":ti,ab or sociocultural:ti,ab	19,504
5	3 AND 4	8047
6	'superwoman schema':ti,ab or 'strong black woman schema':ti,ab or 'Stereotypic Roles for Black Women Scale':ti,ab or SRBWS:ti,ab or SBW:ti,ab or 'Strong Black Women race gender schema':ti,ab	413

(continued on next page)

Set #		Results
	(continued)	
	or 'African American Women s Shifting Scale':ti,ab or AAWSS:ti,ab or 'Strong Black Woman Cultural Construct Scale':ti,ab or SBWCCS:ti,ab or 'Gendered Racial Macroaggressions Scale':ti,ab or GRMS:ti,ab or 'Belgrave Gender Role Inventory':ti,ab or BGRI:ti,ab or 'gender role beliefs':ti,ab or 'gender role belief':ti,ab	
7	5 OR 6	8406
	1 and 2 and 7	324

Database: CINAHL (via EBSCO)

Set #		Results
1	(MH "Blacks") OR TI ("African American" or "African American" or "African Americans" or "African Americans" or Black or Blacks) OR AB ("African American" or "African American" or "African Americans" or "African Americans" or Black or Blacks)	86,478
2	(MH "Women+") OR (MH "Female") OR (MH "Mothers+") OR TI (female or females or womans or women or woman or women's or womens or wife or wives or mother or mothers or daughter or daughters) OR AB (female individual or female individuals or womans or women or woman or women's or womens or wife or wives or mother or mothers or daughter or daughters)	2,116,265
3	(MH "Surveys+") OR (MH "Questionnaires+") OR TI (Schema or schemas or scale or scales or framework or frameworks or questionnaire or questionnaires or inventory or inventories or survey or surveys or tool or tools or measure or measures) OR AB (Schema or schemas or scale or scales or framework or frameworks or questionnaire or questionnaires or inventory or inventories or survey or surveys or tool or tools or measure or measures)	412,026
4	TI ("strong black woman" or "strong black" or superwoman or "super woman" or "stereotypical role" or "stereotypical roles" or "gender role" or "gender roles" or "gendered racism" or "gendered racial" or sociocultural) OR AB ("strong black woman" or "strong black" or superwoman or "super woman" or "stereotypical role" or "stereotypical roles" or "gender role" or "gender roles" or "gendered racism" or "gendered racial" or sociocultural)	6534
5	3 AND 4	1191
6	TI ("superwoman schema" or "strong black woman schema" or "Stereotypic Roles for Black Women Scale" or SRBWS or SBW or "Strong Black Women race gender schema" or "African American Women s Shifting Scale" or AAWSS or "Strong Black Woman Cultural Construct Scale" or SBWCCS or "Gendered Racial Macroaggressions Scale" or GRMS or "Belgrave Gender Role Inventory" or BGRI or "gender role beliefs" or "gender role belief") OR AB TI ("superwoman schema" or "strong black woman schema" or "Stereotypic Roles for Black Women Scale" or SRBWS or SBW or "Strong Black Women race gender schema" or "African American Women s Shifting Scale" or AAWSS or "Strong Black Woman Cultural Construct Scale" or SBWCCS or "Gendered Racial	140

(continued on next page)

(continued)		
Set #		**Results**
	Macroaggressions Scale" or GRMS or "Belgrave Gender Role Inventory" or BGRI or "gender role beliefs" or "gender role belief")	
7	5 OR 6	1310
8	1 and 2 and 7	131

Database: PsycINFO (via EBSCO)

Set #		**Results**
1	DE "Blacks" OR TI ("African American" or "African American" or "African Americans" or "African Americans" or black or blacks) OR AB ("African American" or "African American" or "African Americans" or "African Americans" or black or blacks)	105,288
2	(DE "Human Females") OR (DE "Mothers") OR TI (female individual or female individuals or womans or women or woman or women's or womens or wife or wives or mother or mothers or daughter or daughters) OR AB (female individual or female individuals or womans or women or woman or women's or womens or wife or wives or mother or mothers or daughter or daughters)	677,301
3	(DE "Surveys") OR (DE "Questionnaires") OR TI (Schema or schemas or scale or scales or framework or frameworks or questionnaire or questionnaires or inventory or inventories or survey or surveys or tool or tools or measure or measures) OR AB (Schema or schemas or scale or scales or framework or frameworks or questionnaire or questionnaires or inventory or inventories or survey or surveys or tool or tools or measure or measures)	1,397,780
4	TI ("strong black woman" or "strong black" or superwoman or "super woman" or "stereotypical role" or "stereotypical roles" or "gender role" or "gender roles" or "gendered racism" or "gendered racial" or sociocultural) OR AB ("strong black woman" or "strong black" or superwoman or "super woman" or "stereotypical role" or "stereotypical roles" or "gender role" or "gender roles" or "gendered racism" or "gendered racial" or sociocultural)	27,567
5	3 and 4	9956
6	TI ("superwoman schema" or "strong black woman schema" or "Stereotypic Roles for Black Women Scale" or SRBWS or SBW or "Strong Black Women race gender schema" or "African American Women s Shifting Scale" or AAWSS or "Strong Black Woman Cultural Construct Scale" or SBWCCS or "Gendered Racial Macroaggressions Scale" or GRMS or "Belgrave Gender Role Inventory" or BGRI or "gender role beliefs" or "gender role belief") OR AB ("superwoman schema" or "strong black woman schema" or "Stereotypic Roles for Black Women Scale" or SRBWS or SBW or "Strong Black Women race gender schema" or "African American Women s Shifting Scale" or AAWSS or "Strong Black Woman Cultural Construct Scale" or SBWCCS or "Gendered Racial Macroaggressions Scale" or GRMS or "Belgrave Gender Role Inventory" or BGRI or "gender role beliefs" or "gender role belief")	412
7	5 or 6	10,207
8	1 and 2 and 7	434

Obesity Management in Women

Henry Bohler Jr, MD, MSc

KEYWORDS

- Obesity • Overweight • Adipose tissue • Ultraprocessed foods • Sugar

KEY POINTS

- Obesity is a chronic, relapsing, multifactorial disease.
- The reproductive potential of women and menopause are complicated by obesity.
- Creating a negative energy balance is a key element in the treatment of obesity.
- Diet, physical activity, and most likely, medications are required for prolonged weight reduction.

INTRODUCTION

Obesity is a disease of excess adipose tissue and a wellspring of other conditions such as diabetes, hypertension, stroke, cancer, sleep apnea, osteoarthritis, and depression[1] (**Box 1**). Ultimately, lifespan decreases in parallel with severity.[2] The prevalence of obesity reached epidemic proportions in the United States beginning between 1976 and 1980.[3] Presently, 42% of adults are obese, while 30% are considered overweight. Worldwide, 43% of adults are overweight, while 16% are obese. Among the pediatric population, 35% are either overweight or obese.[4]

Women have higher rates of obesity than men and are more stigmatized when it comes to employment and health care.[5,6] When obesity is present, there is a greater rate of early pubertal development and disrupted menstrual cycles.[6] Polycystic ovarian syndrome, the most common endocrinopathy in women, is frequently precipitated by obesity, which intensifies its signs and symptoms including anovulation, abnormal uterine bleeding, and insulin resistance.[6,7] Obesity also complicates reproduction. Miscarriages, gestational diabetes, and pregnancy-induced hypertension are increased.[6] Endometrial cancer and breast cancer rates are more prevalent in women with obesity.[6,8]

Obesity is not a lack of willpower or a sign of laziness. Its classification as a disease has been endorsed by the Center for Disease Control (CDC), the World Health

Obstetrics and Gynecology, Alum of the University of Louisville, 252 Whittington Parkway, Louisville, KY 40222, USA
E-mail address: henrybohler@gmail.com

Nurs Clin N Am 59 (2024) 593–609
https://doi.org/10.1016/j.cnur.2024.08.005
0029-6465/24/© 2024 Elsevier Inc. All rights reserved, including those for text and data mining, AI training, and similar technologies.

Box 1
Consequences of obesity

- Type 2 diabetes
- Hypertension
- Heart disease
- Sleep apnea
- Fatty liver
- Abnormal lipid profile
- Gall bladder disease
- Arthritis
- Sexual dysfunction
- Fatigue
- Depression
- Cancer
- Alzheimer's disease
- Decreased lifespan

Organization (WHO), and the American Medical Association.[9] But only 1% of physicians treat obesity and most medical schools in the United States consider obesity education a low priority.[10,11] Consequently, providers are neither adequately trained nor feel comfortable addressing patients who are overweight. Additionally, many of the medications that effectively diminish excess adiposity are not covered by insurance, and some of the most effective medications are cost prohibitive.[12] More education is needed to understand the causes, consequences, and current therapies to treat and prevent excess adiposity. With adequate treatment obesity and its comorbidities may be decreased or eradicated.

Adipose Tissue Is Important

Adipose tissue or fat cells and its supportive tissue have several important functions. Fat is our primary source of energy. It provides thermal insulation and cushions our bodies against trauma. It is important in immune and reproduction function and is a source of a myriad of hormones, making it one of the largest endocrine glands in the body.[7] Fat cells secrete leptin, a hormone whose discovery was one of the first clues that food consumption is actively regulated, and not a passive event. Leptin signals the brain that energy stores are sufficient or insufficient for physiologic tasks.[13]

Energy Homeostasis and the Regulation of Fat Stores

Food/energy consumption

Energy homeostasis is the balance between energy consumption (food and drink) and energy expenditure (the amount of energy burned or used).[1] Hunger (an "urgent" need for food) and satiety (a feeling of fullness) are not conscious sensations, but feelings driven by hormonal signals from the gastrointestinal (GI) tract to the central nervous system.[14] The "hunger hormone," ghrelin, is synthesized in the fundus of the stomach, secreted when the stomach is empty and deflated, and activates areas in the brain to cause the sensation of hunger. Ghrelin levels decline after eating and stomach inflation.[14] When nutrients are sensed, peptide YY, cholecystokinin, insulin and glucagon-like peptide-1 (GLP-1), the "satiety hormones," are released from the GI tract and travel to the brain to dock with their receptors.[14] Long-term energy levels are reported by leptin, which is in direct proportion to fat mass and secreted by fat cells.[14] Leptin levels are high in obesity, but due to a "leptin resistance," its signal to reduce caloric intake appears to be blunted.[15]

Energy expenditure
The other half of energy homeostasis is the food or energy expended or burnt, accounted for by the resting metabolic rate (70%), which is influenced by genetics, body mass, age, gender, and climate. This is the energy required to carry out metabolic functions.[16] Physical activity is another 20% (but varies) and includes planned exercise and activity not planned, also called nonexercise activity thermogenesis (NEAT). NEAT includes fidgeting, walking, singing, and so forth and can be substantial, accounting for hundreds of calories burned.[16] NEAT is a possible explanation for why some people curiously remain thin despite their increased calorie consumption.[17] The final 10% of energy used results from diet-induced thermogenesis, the energy needed for digestion, absorption, and storage of food.[18] This may also be referred to as the thermic effect of food (TEF). Each of these components may vary depending on the individual. The TEF may vary depending on the macronutrients digested. For example, protein is more difficult to digest and requires more energy, compared to carbohydrates and fats.[18]

Causes of Obesity

Obesity is a chronic, relapsing, multifactorial disease.[19] Several factors are responsible for the presence of obesity, including genetics, the "obesogenic environment," the quantity and nature of the food consumed, medications, inadequate physical activity, stress, sleep deprivation, as well as hedonic and emotional food consumption.[19]

Genetics
Genetics influences body mass index (BMI) in the range of 40% to 70%, making some individuals more susceptible to weight gain through several polygenic pathways including appetite regulation and basal metabolism.[1,20] This has been demonstrated clearly in studies of children having a similar BMI as their biological parents, despite being adopted and raised in a different environment.[21] Identical twins separated at birth have a 70% chance of having a similar BMI.[21] While BMI may be influenced by multiple genes, there are rare single gene mutations that lead to a dramatic accumulation of excess body fat, usually presenting in early childhood.[1]

The obesogenic environment
Genetic and epigenetic (heritable changes that affect gene function but do not modify DNA sequence) changes occur too slowly to explain the obesity pandemic, which is projected to affect over 3 billion people worldwide by 2030.[22] The increase in the prevalence of obesity has been attributed to our newly acquired "obesogenic environment": not only more food consumption but also an increase in calorie-dense hyperpalatable foods, along with a decrease in physical activity.[23] Increased portion sizes and ingestive frequency factor into a mostly positive energy balance.[24,25]

Sugar and ultraprocessed foods
What is eaten is a major contributor to excess adiposity and much of the blame has been attributed to an excess of sugar intake.[3] Sugar affects the brain reward system and leads to overconsumption. Sugar is a large part of food processing, including

sugar-sweetened beverages, which have contributed to the global epidemic of obesity and cardiometabolic diseases.[3]

All foods are processed (removing unwanted parts, washing, and so forth), but ultra-processed foods (UPFs) refer to industrial processing and added ingredients such as sugar, oils and fats, and salt, making the food hyperpalatable. Sausage, potato chips, and pasta are examples of UPFs. UPFs are not as filling. Not surprisingly, UPFs account for the most calories consumed in the American diet, in part because they are more convenient, like fast foods or frozen dinners. There is less suppression of ghrelin and a diminished release of the satiety hormones, compared to whole foods, which contain no added ingredients and are more nutritious than UPFs.[3]

Stress and sleep deprivation

Stress may be associated with obesity in a variety of ways, including overeating and consumption of calorie-dense "comfort" foods, less physical activity, and shortening sleep.[26,27] Perceived stress increases the secretion of cortisol, which promotes eating, resistance to leptin signals, and abdominal fat accumulation.[27]

Sleep deprivation is independently associated with obesity. In 2021, about 40% of adults reported a decrease in sleeping hours.[28] Less than 7 hours of sleep is associated with increased ghrelin levels, lowered leptin levels and decreased metabolism.[29] An inadequate amount of sleep also leads to a tendency to seek calorie-dense foods.[30]

Obesity increases the risk of obstructive sleep apnea (OSA), found in 24% of men, and 9% of women. Less oxygen is consumed during sleep because of recurrent episodes of complete or partial obstruction of the upper airway. Daytime sleepiness and less physical activity may result. To make matters worse, continuous positive airway pressure has been associated with weight gain, not weight loss.[31]

Medications

Many medications are associated with weight gain, which is often overlooked by the well-intended provider.[32] Many but not all the medications in the following categories have been shown to increase weight significantly: antihypertensives, antidiabetes medications (especially insulin or insulin secretagogues, not metformin), antidepressants, mood stabilizers, migraine medications (not topiramate) antipsychotics, chemotherapeutic agents, antiseizure medications, and hormones, like glucocorticoids and possibly injectable or implantable progestins. Some of these may be avoided and substituted with other medications with either less or no effect on weight or another medication may be added to mitigate the effects of increased fat.[32]

Physical inactivity

Sedentary behavior is a modern-day problem with the advent of electronic devices and less physical locomotion.[33] There is an increase in the prevalence of physical inactivity and sedentary behavior in the obese population.[33]

The menopause transition, a special situation

Transitioning into menopause (perimenopause) is usually heralded by irregular menstrual cycles, hot flashes, night sweats, and disrupted sleep.[34] During this period, there is a change in body composition, with an increase in abdominal fat (subcutaneous and visceral fat) and a decrease in lean body mass (including muscle mass), along with a decline in physical activity and resting energy expenditure.[34,35] Visceral fat accumulation elevates the risk of metabolic disease and may be assumed in with an increase in abdominal waist circumference (WC) due to abdominal subcutaneous fat increases.[34] A drop in estrogen levels may account for a significant part of these changes.[34]

Assessment of Overweight or Obese Patients

Excess adiposity is a highly sensitive topic, and if the provider is broaching the subject (and not the patient), it must be done with sensitivity. There is a blueprint to go by and it is called the 5 As.[36] The first may be the most important. Ask for permission to discuss his or her weight.[36] Sample questions from Sandra Christensen of the Obesity Medical Association: "Do I have your permission to discuss your weight? Would you be willing to discuss your weight? Do you have any concerns about your weight?"[18] The rest of the As include assess, advise, agree, and assist.[36] Avoid words like "fat" and "obese."

If weight management is the presenting concern, almost all have tried to lose weight previously, usually by dieting, sometimes with the addition of medications, and occasionally with bariatric surgery. It is helpful to know what worked before. Those with a history of bariatric surgery should have appropriate follow-up to exclude micronutrient deficiencies.[18] In brief, body weight history, nutrition history, sleep history, medical history, family history, social history medications, and review of systems should be done (**Boxes 2–4, Table 1**). Details may be found in the Obesity Algorithm published by the Obesity Medicine Association.[18,37]

Box 2
Weight and nutrition history

Age and gender

Present weight and height

Age of onset of weight gain

Greatest weight

Desired weight

Weight increased over: years or months

Weight gain started because of
- Decreased activity
- Stress
- Marriage/*divorce*
- Illness
- New job
- Pregnancy
- Menopause
- Relocation
- Retirement
- Anxiety
- Depression
- Medications
- Other

Nutritional History: Triggers
- Sweets
- Sweetened beverages
- Multiple snacks
- Nighttime eating (after dinner)
- Experiences cravings
- Boredom
- Binges
- Other

Box 3
Sleep history
Number of hours
Shift work (work at night often)
Snoring
Sleep apnea
Sleepy during the day

Physical examination

Vital signs (especially blood pressure), height, weight, BMI, and neck and waist circumferences should be recorded (**Tables 2** and **3**).[18]

Box 4
Medical history
Prediabetes/diabetes
Gestational diabetes
Polycystic ovary syndrome
Heart disease
High blood pressure
High cholesterol
Thyroid disease or thyroid cancer
MEN2 disease
Osteoarthritis
Kidney disease
Liver disease or fatty liver
Pancreatitis
Gallbladder disease
Gastrointestinal disease
Irritable bowel syndrome
Crohn's disease
Gastric reflux
Chronic fatigue
Fibromyalgia
Anxiety
Depression
Sleep apnea
Easy bruising
Cancer
Other

Table 1
Family history

	Mother	Father	Brother	Sister	Grandparents
Diabetes					
Hypertension					
Increased cholesterol					
Thyroid disease					
Cancer					
Obesity					

Measurements to detect the presence of obesity. The BMI is used to detect excess body fat and is calculated by dividing the weight of an individual in kilograms by their height in meters squared[38] (to get meters, divide the height in centimeters by 100). Thus, it is a surrogate and not a direct measurement for body fatness. It is used because it is easy to measure, and it correlates strongly with body fat quantity and increase in the risk of disease.[38] Direct and more accurate measures of fat quantity with computerized tomography or MRI are impractical and too expensive.[39] A more muscular person, age, sex, and ethnic groups may interfere with the accuracy of BMI in predicting the risk of disease (WHO expert consultation); nevertheless, BMI serves as a good screening tool and is the standard measured in most research articles on obesity. A normal or healthy BMI ranges from 18.5 to 24.9; obesity equals a BMI of 30 or more,[18] while overweight is between a BMI of 25 and 29.9. Comorbid conditions are also found in overweight individuals, including an increase in mortality.[40]

Percent body fat. Percent body fat is another metric to detect adiposity, but normal levels vary depending on reference standards and age (US Army vs American Council on Exercise Classification). It may be especially useful in those who are losing or not losing weight because of increasing muscle mass in the face of less adipose tissue, which might occur with resistance training. Measurements of body fat percentage (BF%) may vary with calipers, electronic devices that use impedance of different tissues, the operator, hydration, and other factors.[41] Dual-energy x-ray absorptiometry scan is the most accurate means of measuring BF%. Greater than or equal to 32% BF is elevated in women; 25% or greater BF is increased in men.[42]

Waist circumference. WC accurately predicts metabolic disease.[43] The Centers for Disease Control and Prevention (CDC) suggest measuring it with a tape measure horizontally applied at the top of the iliac crest, snug after the patient expires.[44] The navel as a landmark will not be consistent since this may vary among individuals. An increase in WC is associated with a rise in intra-abdominal or visceral fat, which is

Table 2
Weight and body mass index

Classification	BMI
Underweight	Below 18.5
Normal weight	18.5–24.9
Overweight (preobese)	25–29.9
Obese	30 or more

Table 3 Waist circumference	
Women	$\geq$35 in or >88 cm
Men	$\geq$40 in or $\geq$102 cm

more strongly correlated with metabolic disturbances than subcutaneous fat.[45] Disease risk increases at a WC of 35 inches or 89 cm or greater for women and 40 inches or 102 cm or greater for men. But this cutoff changes with the population studied. For example, in Asians, the cut point is 31.5 inches (80 cm) or greater for women and 35 inches (89 cm) or greater for men.[46] One study found that an increase in insulin resistance in African American men was found at a WC of 102 cm or greater and for AA women, the cut point was 98 cm or greater.[47] WC may not be a useful adjunct to BMI if the BMI is greater than 35 kg/m^2.[18]

Neck circumference. Neck circumference may also be useful in predicting OSA and metabolic disease. Neck circumference is obtained with a tape measure at the level of the cricothyroid membrane. Greater than 17 inches in men and more than 16 inches in women increase the risk for OSA.[48] OSA should be suspected if there is loud snoring, gasping, and obesity.[48] The rest of the physical examination may be done according to the signs and symptoms of the patient. For example, in a female individual with polycystic ovary syndrome, the presence of insulin resistance may be evident by the finding of hirsutism and/or acanthosis nigricans in the neck area.

Laboratory analysis
Laboratory analysis includes fasting glucose, hemoglobin A1c, fasting lipids, liver enzymes, electrolytes, renal function test, uric acid, thyroid stimulating test, and 25-hydroxyvitamin D levels (**Box 5**). Prediabetes (or diabetes), dyslipidemia, fatty liver, and low vitamin D levels are common conditions found with obesity. Other tests may be appropriate depending on the patient's presentation or test results. For example, testosterone levels may be low in male individuals with low libido and obesity, an electrocardiogram (EKG) with a long history of hypertension and a nocturnal polysomnography for suspected OSA.[18]

Box 5 Laboratory analysis
Fasting blood glucose
Hemoglobin A1c
Fasting lipids: triglycerides, low-density lipoprotein cholesterol, high-density lipoprotein (HDL) cholesterol, and non-HDL cholesterol
Liver enzymes: aspartate aminotransferase, alanine aminotransferase, alkaline phosphatase, and total bilirubin
Electrolytes
Renal blood test (creatinine and blood urea nitrogen)
Uric acid
Thyroid-stimulating hormone
25-hydroxyvitamin D

Management of Excess Adiposity

Address all factors contributing to obesity

Because obesity is a multifactorial disease, all factors contributing to excess food consumption should be addressed. For example, in the presence of sleep deprivation, and maneuvers may be needed to insure a removal of sleep deprivers, like caffeine, alcohol, phone, computer and TV screens. Elements leading to chronic stress should be identified and deleted, if possible; if not counseling or mitigating stress with walking, exercise, meditation, and a restful sleep could be attempted. Consider consulting with the original prescriber of weight-inducing medications.

Diet

Portion control and nutritious eating should be encouraged for not only weight loss but also for better health. Most diets have advantages and disadvantages with no clear winner, whether its low carb, low fat, or high protein. When possible, a nutritionist or dietician involvement is very helpful.

The main ingredient is an energy deficit, no matter the diet. The number of calories restricted can be obtained by calculating the patients' total daily energy requirement (or expenditure; TDER), which factors in their metabolism, weight, height, age, sex, and activity level. This is placed into a readily available formula (based on the Harris Benedict Equation), resulting in the amount of kilocalories per day for female and male individuals.[49] The formula is not perfectly fitted for every individual, and there is variability (eg, variability in metabolism). Theoretically, 500 kcal below the calculated amount may lead to a 1 lb weight loss per week. So, the patient is asked to weigh her or himself at least weekly, if not daily and if not losing weight, subtract more calories (eg, 300 calories more) until this is achieved. The sources to assist with daily calorie intake include food labels that provide calories per serving and apps like MyFitnessPal and Fooducate. Even Siri on an iPhone can help! "Hey Siri, how many calories are there in" my whatever, and it will tell you. This is the initial TDER but it changes as weight decreases. Adjustment can be made at the follow-up visits.

Once the TDER is calculated along with the targeted deficit, prescribe percentages of macronutrients. The United States Department of Agriculture (USDA) recommended percentages is 45% to 65% of your daily calories from carbs, 20% to 35% of your total calories from fats, 10% to 35% of your daily calories from protein for adults not losing weight, but for weight loss, fewer carbs (30%–40% of calories), fat (20%–30% of calories), and more protein (25%–35% of calories) may be beneficial.[50,51] An example of a diet of 1500 kcal/d determined to be the deficit for an individual: Carbohydrates: 40% of 1500 = 600 calories/4 calories per gram = 150 g. The remaining macronutrients are calculated similarly. Protein, 4 kcal/g; fats, 9 kcal/g (**Table 4**).

Nutrition therapy suggested by The Obesity Medical Association includes a low-calorie diet between 1000 and 1200 kcal/d for women and between 1200 and 1600 kcal/d for men. If opting for fat restriction, a low-fat diet would be less than 30% fat; if carbohydrate restricting, less than 26% of total calories or less than 130 g/d.[18] In terms of weight loss, neither is superior.[52]

Table 4 Sample diet based on 1500 C/day			
Calories C/d	Carbs 40% 4 C/g	Fat 25% 9 C/g	Protein 30% 4 C/g
1500	150 g	42 g	131 g

Many patients will not count calories but will start to be mindful of their portions and what they eat or do not eat. It is important that the patient becomes mindful of real "hunger and satiety signals" and not eating without these cues.[53] Whole foods and not UPFs should be consumed as much as possible, on most days. They are more satiating and less calorie dense.

Physical activity

Physical activity or the dreaded word "exercise" clearly has many redeeming qualities: a better sense of well-being, better sleep, an improvement in metabolic parameters, protection from cardiovascular disease, and the list goes on.[18] The patient should be physically fit to engage in an increased activity program as determined by you or another provider and that may include an EKG or other studies, depending on the patient's condition, age, and previous exercise history.[18]

If resistance training is planned, a personal trainer may be helpful to assist with the proper training methods and to prevent injury, especially in older adults. Resistance training (usually weightlifting) should be encouraged because along with adequate protein intake, it may increase muscle mass or at least mitigate muscle atrophy.[54] Twenty percent of lean body mass loss, along with fat loss, is expected with weight reduction from calorie restriction.[55] This is particularly important in older individuals where muscle downsizing with age is the norm along with a drop in basal metabolism.[56] Physical activity often declines with age.

Any activity promotes good health. Walking daily with a goal working toward 10,000 steps a day is beneficial (less than 5000 steps is considered sedentary).[18] Exercise of moderate intensity—150 to 250 minutes per week or at least 75 minutes of vigorous physical activity—aids in preventing weight gain, but not much weight loss.[57] For a more significant amount of weight loss, at least 250 minutes a week of more vigorous physical activity (eg, running, swimming, or singles tennis) is required.[57] A good exercise plan might include aerobic exercise 3 days a week and resistance training at least twice each week.[58] Start with atomic habits.[59] Put the shoes by the door. Ask a friend to join in. Hire a personal trainer and make an appointment that must be kept! Some may be limited in mobility because of accompanying medical conditions, but this may change with a decrease in weight. Encourage physical activity at any level.

Antiobesity medications

The list of antiobesity medications (AOMs) is growing and not all will be discussed here, but there has been a sea change in medications available that effectively thwart the counterregulatory actions aimed to maintain excess adiposity (**Table 5**). Weight loss medications may be used along with diet and physical activity either if the BMI is 30 kg/m^2 or greater or if the BMI is 27 kg/m^2 or greater in the presence of a comorbidity related to weight gain, such as hypertension, diabetes, dyslipidemia, and depression (there are others).[18] Some of the most exciting and effective AOMs include the incretins.[60]

The incretins include glucagon-like peptide-1 (GLP-1) and glucose-dependent insulinotropic polypeptide (GIP).[61,62] They are released from intestinal cells when nutrients are sensed. The use of medications modeled after the incretins has arguably altered the landscape of weight management forever. "Incretins" refers to intestinal-derived factors capable of stimulating the pancreas to release insulin in a glucose-dependent manner.[61,62] Consequently, the chance of hypoglycemia is low, even while using metformin, which partly increases the sensitivity of the cells to insulin.[63] But other glucose-lowering medications, like insulin or the sulfonylureas, should be avoided or used with caution. Lower doses may be necessary to avoid severe hypoglycemia.[64] The incretin class of medications approved for weight loss by the US Food and Drug Administration

Table 5
Commonly used medications

Medication	Effectiveness Weight Reduction	Side Effects (All Are Not Included)	Approved for Long-Term Therapy	Contraindications
Semaglutide Wegovy, (Novo Nortis, Kalundborg, Denmark)(GIP1RA)	10%–17%	Nausea, vomiting, constipation, and diarrhea	Yes	History of medullary thyroid cancer, multiple endocrine neoplasia type 2, suicidal attempts, pregnancy, hypersensitivity, and gastroparesis
Tirzepatide (Zepbound,Eli Lilly and Company, Concord, North Carolina)-GLP1RA/GIPRA	21%	Same as semaglutide	Yes	Same as semaglutide
Phentermine (KVK-Tech, Inc., Newtown, Pennsylvania)	3%–8% t	Increase in blood pressure, heart rate, insomnia, and dry mouth	No	History of cardiovascular disease (CVD), uncontrolled hypertension, during or within 14 d of monoamine oxidase inhibitors (MAOI)use, and alcohol consumption
Topiramate (Topamax,[Janssen Pharmaceuticals, Titusville, New Jersey])	10% May treat binge eating and cravings	Fatigue, memory loss, attention difficulty, tingling, change of taste, depression, suicidal ideation, and risk of cleft lip if taken during pregnancy	Not approved for weight loss	Pregnancy, glaucoma, hyperthyroidism, concomitant MAOI within 14 d, and history of kidney stones
Phentermine/topiramate(Qysmia, Vivus, Inc., Campbell, California)	9% reduction in weight	Numbness, tingling, dizziness, change is taste, and fatigue	Yes	Pregnancy, glaucoma, hyperthyroidism, and concomitant MAOI within 14 d
Naloxone/bupropion (Contrave Currax Pharmaceuticals LLC, Brentwood, Tennessee)	8%–11%	Nausea, constipation, headache, and vomiting	Yes	Uncontrolled hypertension, seizure disorder, discontinuation of alcohol, barbiturates, benzodiazepines, antiepileptics, chronic opioid use, and concomitant MAOI within 14 d
Metformin (Glucophage,Merck KGaA, Darmstadt, Germany)	2%–5%	Gastrointestinal, other	Not approved for weight loss	Renal impairment, metabolic acidosis, and hypersensitivity, before radiologic studies with contrast

(FDA) include Wegovy (semaglutide [SG], GLP-1) (Novo Nordisk, Plainsboro, New Jersey), and Zepbound (tirzepatide, GLP-1, and GIP) (Eli Lilly, Indianapolis, Indiana).[65]

Semaglutide. SG is a glucagon-like peptide receptor agonist (GLP-1RA) similar in structure to the native GLP-1, but has a half-life of 7 days, compared to 2 to 3 minutes for the native hormone.[66] GLP-1 monitors and controls glucose levels by stimulating insulin release (classified as an "incretin") when glucose levels are high, suppressing glucagon release from the pancreas (glucagon increases glucose release from the liver) and by decreasing gastric emptying and glucose absorption.[61] It was originally developed for the treatment of patients with type 2 diabetes in whom weight loss was also observed. In addition to all the aforementioned actions, it increases satiety, through central and peripheral mechanisms and has been FDA approved (Wegovy) for weight loss.[64,65]

With subcutaneous injections, the average weight loss is approximately 15%.[67] Results from SG also include decreased WC, hemoglobin A1c, blood pressure, low-density lipoprotein cholesterol, triglycerides, and, importantly, cardiovascular events, including death, myocardial infarction, and stroke.[68] Side effects are mostly GI, including nausea, vomiting, diarrhea, and constipation, usually transient and not enough to discontinue therapy.[67] Nausea is more likely in the first several weeks of therapy, with monthly dose escalation, decreasing over time. Reducing portion size, eating slowly, and avoiding high-fat meals may be helpful, along with antiemetics, like ondansetron.[64] Despite the reduction in gastric motility, diarrhea may also occur, and it has been posited that this is osmotic owing to a reduced intestinal uptake of glucose and lipids caused by GIP-1RAs.[64] Apparently, metformin in combination with SG may sometimes exacerbate the adverse GI effects.[69] Constipation can be treated by increasing fruit, fiber, and water intake. A complete list of untoward effects will not be listed here, but gallbladder disease (possibly from a rapid weight loss), acute pancreatitis and an exacerbation of diabetic retinopathy are sighted as possible consequences of therapy.[64] Contraindications include a history of medullary thyroid cancer or multiple endocrine neoplasia type 2 (MEN2).[64] AOMs should not be taken during pregnancy.[70]

Because of possible side effects, doses are escalated gradually, approximately doubling each month starting with 0.25 mg, 0.5 mg, 1 mg, 1.7 mg, and finally 2.4 mg, with subcutaneous injections in the thigh, abdomen, or upper arm.[71] Once the target weight is reached, the medication may be stopped suddenly or titrated downward. With lifestyle changes, including better eating habits, increasing physical activity, and improved sleep, discontinuing the medication is possible. But increased hunger and appetite most likely will occur. Presently, there is no time limit to continue either incretin for obesity, just as there are no time constraints for medical treatments for other chronic diseases, like diabetes and hypertension. Patients should be monitored for effectiveness of therapy and untoward effects.

Tirzepatide. Tirzepatide (TZ) combines 2 intestinal incretin agonists, GLP-1 and GIP. Zepbound (tirzepatide) has been FDA approved for weight loss.[65] Weight reductions on average were 20% at the maximum dose, which is reached with monthly dose escalations of 2.5 mg until the maximum dose of 15 mg is reached. It is more effective than SG on average.[72] Beyond weight reduction, other cardiovascular and metabolic factors were improved, such as WC, blood pressure, hemoglobin A1 c, lipids, and liver enzymes.[73] More fat than lean body mass was reduced. Side effects are like SG.

Presently, SG and TZ may cost at least US$1500 each month.

Phentermine. Low cost, effective, and tolerable side effects make phentermine an acceptable initial medication and is the most used medication for weight loss in the

United States. Average weight reduction is 3% to 8%.[74] Like all weight loss medications, it decreases appetite, with its primary effects in the central nervous system.[74] It is a stimulant; therefore, it should be taken in the very early hours of the day to avoid insomnia. Blood pressure and pulse rate should be monitored, but it may be given to patients with controlled hypertension. Available doses vary and taken in divided doses or once a day.[74]

Phentermine is listed as a schedule IV drug and is structurally like amphetamines, but its potential for abuse is low.[74] Nevertheless, it is recommended that phentermine be used for no more than 3 months and avoided in those with a history of drug abuse. It should also be avoided in patients using monoamine oxidase inhibitors, cardiovascular disease, hyperthyroidism, and glaucoma.[74] Other side effects include dry mouth and jitteriness.[74] When combined with topiramate, it is approved for long-term use.

Topiramate. Topiramate as monotherapy is not FDA-approved for weight loss but some have used it "off label." It is more commonly used for migraine headaches and seizure disorders, for which it is approved. As much as 6% to 16% weight reduction may be expected.[75] It is effective for cravings and binge eating.[76] Topiramate acts on the central nervous system, decreasing appetite. Side effects include but are not limited to paresthesia (tingling in the extremities), fatigue, memory loss, and a change of taste (sodas are not as tasty). It may also increase the risk of kidney stones, myopia, and angle glaucoma.[18]

Phentermine and topiramate. Phentermine and topiramate have been combined into one drug and is listed as a schedule IV medication. As much as 10% weight loss can be expected. The warnings and contraindications are the same as for the individual drugs used as monotherapy. It has been approved for long-term use along with SG and tirzepatide.

SUMMARY

Obesity is a disease much like any other chronic disease with multiple causes. Therefore, all contributing factors should be addressed to assist in effective weight loss. Weight reduction is challenging, in part, because of metabolic adaptations and hormonal changes that favor weight regain, and these changes persist for months, if not years.[77,78] Creating an energy deficit is the core of effective treatment of obesity. Physical activity is especially important to maintain weight reduction. Medications have an important role in reducing food consumption, unless contraindicated.

CLINICS CARE POINTS

- Obesity is not due to a lack of willpower.
- It should be approached with sensitivity and managed after the patient's consent.
- The diagnosis of overweight and obesity is made by obtaining the body mass index but waist circumference is equally, if not more important during the assessment.
- Because of physiologic adaptations to diet and exercise, medications are important adjuncts to effective therapy for weight loss.
- Patients should be encouraged to maintain their prescribed diet and activity and monitored for effectiveness and side effects resulting from management.
- Body weight may plateau regardless of the type of intervention.

DECLARATION OF AI AND AI-ASSISTED TECHNOLOGIES IN THE WRITING PROCESS

During the preparation of this article the author(s) used Perplexity AI in order to assist in a general outline of this chapter as well as to investigate information further. After using this tool/service, the author reviewed and edited the content as needed and takes full responsibility for the content of the publication.

DISCLOSURE

The authors have no disclosures.

REFERENCES

1. Steven B, Heymsfield MD, Wadden Thomas A. Mechanisms, pathophysiology, and management of obesity. N Engl J Med 2017;376:254–66.
2. Khan S, Ning H, Wilkins JT, et al. Association of body mass index with lifetime risk of cardiovascular disease and compression of morbidity. JAMA Cardiol 2018; 3(4):280–7.
3. Temple NJ. The origins of the obesity epidemic in the USA-lessons for today. Nutrients 2022;14(20):4253.
4. Overweight and obesity statistics. Available at: niddk.nih.gov. Accessed April 6, 2024.
5. Kapoor N, Arora S, Kalra S. Gender disparities in people living with obesity - an unchartered territory. J Mid-life Health 2021;12:103–7.
6. Link DG. Obesity in women: paying a high price. Nurs Clin N Am 2021;56:609–17.
7. Bohler H Jr, Mokshagundam S, Winters SJ. Adipose tissue and reproduction in women. Fertil Steril 2010;94(3):795–825.
8. Crafts TD, Tonneson JE, Wolfe BM, et al. Obesity and breast cancer: preventive and therapeutic possibilities for bariatric surgery. Obesity 2022;30(3):587–98.
9. Kyle TK, Dhurandhar EJ, Allison DB. Regarding obesity as a disease: evolving policies and their implications. Endocrinol Metab Clin North Am 2016;45(3): 511–20.
10. Gudzune KA, Johnson VR, Bramante CT, et al. Geographic availability of physicians certified by the American Board of Obesity medicine relative to obesity prevalence. Obesity 2019;27(12):1958–66.
11. Butsch WS, Kushner RF, Alford S, et al. Low priority of obesity education leads to lack of medical students' preparedness to effectively treat patients with obesity: results from the U.S. medical school obesity education curriculum benchmark study. BMC Med Educ 2020;20(1):23.
12. Reitman E. Anti-obesity medication's steep price tag adds to public health disparities. Available at: medicine.yale.edu. Accessed July 30, 2024.
13. Cypess AM. Reassessing human adipose tissue. N Engl J Med 2022;386(8): 768–79.
14. Tack J, Verbeure W, Mori H, et al. The gastrointestinal tract in hunger and satiety signalling. United European Gastroenterol J 2021;9(6):727–34.
15. Liu J, Yang X, Yu S, et al. The leptin resistance. Adv Exp Med Biol 2018;1090: 145–63, 30390289.
16. Moehlecke M, Canani L, Oliveira L, et al. Determinants of body weight regulation in humans. Arch Endocrinol Metab 2016;60(2):152–62.
17. Chung N, Park MY, Kim J, et al. Non-exercise activity thermogenesis (NEAT): a component of total daily energy expenditure. J Exerc Nutrition Biochem 2018; 22(2):23–30.

18. Tondt J, Freshwater M, Christensen S, et al. Obesity algorithm ebook, presented by the obesity medicine association. www.obesityalgorithm.org. 2023. https://obesitymedicine.org (Accessed April 6, 2024).

19. Lin X, Li H. Obesity: epidemiology, pathophysiology, and therapeutics. Front Endocrinol 2021;12:706978.

20. Bray MS, Loos RJ, McCaffery JM, et al. NIH working group report-using genomic information to guide weight management: from universal to precision treatment. Obesity 2016;24:14–22.

21. Maes HH, Neale MC, Eaves LJ. Genetic and environmental factors in relative body weight and human adiposity. Behav Genet 1997;27(4):325–51.

22. Herrera BM, Keildson S, Lindgren CM. Genetics and epigenetics of obesity. Maturitas 2011;69(1):41–9.

23. Nicolaidis S. Environment and obesity. Metabolism 2019;100S:153942.

24. Livingstone MB, Pourshahidi LK. Portion size and obesity. Adv Nutr 2014;5(6):829–34.

25. Mattes R. Energy intake and obesity: ingestive frequency outweighs portion size. Physiol Behav 2014;134:110–8.

26. Dallman MF, Pecoraro N, Akana SF, et al. Chronic stress and obesity: a new view of "comfort food". Proc Natl Acad Sci U S A 2003;100(20):11696–701.

27. Tomiyama AJ. Stress and obesity. Annu Rev Psychol 2019;70:703–18.

28. Sleep and sleep disorders. Available at: CDC.gov. Accessed April 6, 2024.

29. Chaput JP, McHill AW, Cox RC, et al. The role of insufficient sleep and circadian misalignment in obesity. Nat Rev Endocrinol 2023;19(2):82–97.

30. Papatriantafyllou E, Efthymiou D, Zoumbaneas E, et al. Sleep deprivation: effects on weight loss and weight loss maintenance. Nutrients 2022;14(8):1549.

31. Redenius R, Murphy C, O'Neill E, et al. Does CPAP lead to change in BMI? J Clin Sleep Med 2008;4(3):205–9.

32. Singh S, Ricardo-Silgado ML, Bielinski SJ, et al. Pharmacogenomics of medication-induced weight gain and antiobesity medications. Obesity 2021;29(2):265–73.

33. Silveira EA, Mendonça CR, Delpino FM, et al. Sedentary behavior, physical inactivity, abdominal obesity and obesity in adults and older adults: a systematic review and meta-analysis. Clin Nutr ESPEN 2022;50:63–73.

34. Marlatt KL, Pitynski-Miller DR, Gavin KM, et al. Body composition and cardiometabolic health across the menopause transition. Obesity 2022;30(1):14–27.

35. Greendale GA, Sternfeld B, Huang M, et al. Changes in body composition and weight during the menopause transition. JCI Insight 2019;4(5):e124865.

36. Wharton S, et al. CMAJ (Can Med Assoc J) 2020;192(31):E875–91.

37. Elmaleh-Sachs A, Schwartz JL, Bramante CT, et al. Obesity management in adults: a review. JAMA 2023;330(20):2000–15.

38. Overweight and obesity. Available at: CDC.gov. Accessed August 29, 2023.

39. What is the Gold Standard for Determining Body Fat. 2023. Available at: https://obesitymedicine.org. (Accessed 2 August 2024).

40. Wyatt SB, Winters KP, Dubbert PM. Overweight and obesity: prevalence, consequences, and causes of a growing public health problem. Am J Med Sci 2006;331(4):166–74.

41. Kuriyan R. Body composition techniques. Indian J Med Res 2018;148(5):648–58.

42. Body Fat Percentage: Charting Averages in Men and Women. Available at: Acefitness.org. (Accessed 13 November 2023).

43. Ross R, Neeland IJ, Yamashita S, et al. Waist circumference as a vital sign in clinical practice: a consensus statement from the IAS and ICCR working group on visceral obesity. Nat Rev Endocrinol 2020;16(3):177–89.

44. Healthy weight, nutrition and physical activity. Available at: CDC.gov. Accessed April 6, 2024.

45. Boone SC, van Smeden M, Rosendaal FR, et al. Evaluation of the value of waist circumference and metabolomics in the estimation of visceral adipose tissue. Am J Epidemiol 2022;191(5):886–99.

46. Camhi SM, Bray GA, Bouchard C, et al. The relationship of waist circumference and BMI to visceral, subcutaneous, and total body fat: sex and race differences. Obesity 2011;19(2):402–8.

47. Sumner AE, Sen S, Ricks M, et al. Determining the waist circumference in African Americans which best predicts insulin resistance. Obesity 2008;16(4):841–6.

48. Semelka M, Wilson J, Floyd R. Diagnosis and treatment of obstructive sleep apnea in adults. Am Fam Physician 2016;94(5):355–60.

49. In Epocrates Drug/Disease Clinical Support for Apple iOS (Version 24.7) [Mobile application software].

50. Available at: http://www.usda.gov/guidance. (Accessed 6 April 2024).

51. The Best Macronutrient Ratio for Weight Loss. Available at: https://www.medicine.net.com. (Accessed 25 March 2024).

52. Sacks FM, Bray GA, Carey VJ, et al. Comparison of weight-loss diets with different compositions of fat, protein, and carbohydrates. N Engl J Med 2009;360(9):859–73.

53. Available at: https://www.health.harvard.edu. (Accessed 5 April 2024).

54. He N, Ye H. Exercise and muscle atrophy. Adv Exp Med Biol 2020;1228:255–67.

55. Pasiakos SM, Cao JJ, Margolis LM, et al. Effects of high-protein diets on fat-free mass and muscle protein synthesis following weight loss: a randomized controlled trial. FASEB J 2013;27(9):3837–47.

56. Fry CS, Rasmussen BB. Skeletal muscle protein balance and metabolism in the elderly. Curr Aging Sci 2011;4(3):260–8.

57. Donnelly JE, Blair SN, Jakicic JM, et al, American College of Sports Medicine. American College of Sports Medicine Position Stand. Appropriate physical activity intervention strategies for weight loss and prevention of weight regain for adults. Med Sci Sports Exerc 2009;41(2):459–71 [Erratum appears in Med Sci Sports Exerc. 2009;41(7):1532].

58. Adult Activity Available at: An Overview.cdc.gov/physical-activity-basics/guidelines/adults.html. (Accessed 27 March 2004).

59. Clear J. Atomic Habits: an easy and proven way to build good habits and break bad ones. New York: Avery: PDF edition; 2018.

60. Rehfeld JF. The origin and understanding of the incretin concept. Front Endocrinol 2018;9:387.

61. Baggio LL, Drucker DJ. Biology of incretins: GLP-1 and GIP. Gastroenterology 2007;132(6):2131–57.

62. Campbell JE, Drucker DJ. Pharmacology, physiology, and mechanisms of incretin hormone action. Cell Metabol 2013;17(6):819–37.

63. Korsatko S, Jensen L, Brunner M, et al. Effect of once-weekly semaglutide on the counterregulatory response to hypoglycaemia in people with type 2 diabetes: a randomized, placebo-controlled, double-blind, crossover trial. Diabetes Obes Metabol 2018;20(11):2565–73.

64. Smits MM, Van Raalte DH. Safety of semaglutide. Front Endocrinol 2021;12:645563.

65. FDA Approves New Drug/Medication Treatment for Chronic Weight Management. Available at: @https://www.fda.gov.gov (Accessed 7 April 2024).

66. Hall S, Isaacs D, Clements JN. Pharmacokinetics and clinical implications of semaglutide: a new glucagon-like peptide (GLP)-1 receptor agonist. Clin Pharmacokinet 2018;57(12):1529–38.

67. Garvey WT, Batterham RL, Bhatta M, et al, STEP 5 Study Group. Two-year effects of semaglutide in adults with overweight or obesity: the STEP 5 trial. Nat Med 2022;28(10):2083–91.

68. Lincoff AM, Brown-Frandsen K, Colhoun HM, et al. SELECT trial investigators. semaglutide and cardiovascular outcomes in obesity without diabetes. N Engl J Med 2023;389(24):2221–32.

69. Bettge K, Kahle M, Abd El Aziz MS, et al. Occurrence of nausea, vomiting and diarrhoea reported as adverse events in clinical trials studying glucagon-like peptide-1 receptor agonists: a systematic analysis of published clinical trials. Diabetes Obes Metabol 2017;19(3):336–47.

70. Muller DRP, Stenvers DJ, Malekzadeh A, et al. Effects of GLP-1 agonists and SGLT2 inhibitors during pregnancy and lactation on offspring outcomes: a systematic review of the evidence. Front Endocrinol 2023;14:1215356.

71. Wilding JPH, Batterham RL, Calanna S, et al, STEP 1 Study Group. Once-weekly semaglutide in adults with overweight or obesity. N Engl J Med 2021;384(11):989–1002.

72. Azuri J, Hammerman A, Aboalhasan E, et al. Tirzepatide versus semaglutide for weight loss in patients with type 2 diabetes mellitus: a value for money analysis. Diabetes Obes Metabol 2023;25(4):961–4.

73. Rosenstock J, Wysham C, Frías JP, et al. Efficacy and safety of a novel dual GIP and GLP-1 receptor agonist tirzepatide in patients with type 2 diabetes (SUR-PASS-1): a double-blind, randomised, phase 3 trial. Lancet 2021;398(10295):143–55.

74. Bays HE, Lazarus E, Primack C, et al. Obesity pillars roundtable: phentermine - Past, present, and future. Obes Pillars 2022;3:100024. PMID: 37990729; PMCID: PMC10661986.

75. Verrotti A, Scaparrotta A, Agostinelli S, et al. Topiramate-induced weight loss: a review. Epilepsy Res 2011;95(3):189–99.

76. Tata AL, Kockler DR. Topiramate for binge-eating disorder associated with obesity. Ann Pharmacother 2006;40(11):1993–7.

77. Martins C, Gower BA, Hunter GR. Metabolic adaptation delays time to reach weight loss goals. Obesity 2022;30(2):400–6.

78. Sumithran P, Prendergast LA, Delbridge E, et al. Long-term persistence of hormonal adaptations to weight loss. N Engl J Med 2011;365(17):1597–604. PMID: 22029981.

Nursing Process Approach to Pain Management for Women with Polysubstance Use

Derrick C. Glymph, PhD, DNAP, CRNA, CHSE, CNE, COL, USAR[a],*,
Rishelle Y. Zhou, DNAP, LLB, CRNA[b],
Daniel D. King, DNP, MNA, CRNA, APRN, CPPS, CNE[c],
Tamar Rodney, PhD, RN, PMHNP-BC, CNE[d]

KEYWORDS

• Substance use disorder • Women • Pain management • Nursing process

KEY POINTS

• There is a complex intersection of chronic pain and substance use disorder (SUD) in women, which presents multifaceted challenges.
• The nursing process as a guiding framework provides an evidenced-based systematic approach to planning across the continuum of care.
• An interdisciplinary multimodal approach should include pharmacologic and non-pharmacologic interventions.
• A tailored intervention and shared decision-making approach to pain management for women with SUD is vital.

INTRODUCTION

Pain is a complex and unpleasant experience associated with actual or potential tissue damage.[1,2] Acute pain is associated with sudden onset and a limited duration of 1 month or less.[3] Acute pain can often evolve into chronic pain, which typically lasts more than 3 months. Data from the National Health Interview Survey in 2019 demonstrate that, in the United States (US), approximately 1 in 5 adults has chronic pain and

---

[a] Nurse Anesthesia Program, Duke University School of Nursing, 307 Trent Drive, DUMC 3037, Durham, NC 27710, USA; [b] Nurse Anesthesia Program, VA Portland Health Care System, Oregon Health and Science University School of Nursing, 97239 /3455 Southwest US Veterans Hospital Road, 3710 Southwest US Veterans Hospital Road, Portland, OR 97239, USA; [c] Nurse Anesthesia Program, Rosalind Franklin University of Medicine and Science, College of Nursing, 3333 Green Bay Road, North Chicago, IL 60064-3095, USA; [d] Johns Hopkins University School of Nursing, 525 North Wolfe Street, Baltimore, MD 21205, USA
* Corresponding author.
E-mail address: Derrick.glymph@duke.edu

Nurs Clin N Am 59 (2024) 611–624
https://doi.org/10.1016/j.cnur.2024.08.002   **nursing.theclinics.com**

1 in 14 adults is affected by high-impact pain.[4] High-impact chronic pain is defined as pain that causes limited work and life activities almost every day or most days over a 3-month period.[4,5] The survey showed that women were more likely to suffer from chronic pain (21.7%) compared to men (19%) (**Fig. 1**).[5,6] It also demonstrated that the prevalence of high-impact pain was higher among women (8.5%) compared to men (7.4%).[2–4] Treating chronic pain can be difficult as chronic pain is affected by the complex nervous system and multidimensional factors such as mental health, hormonal fluctuation, emotions, and other health conditions. Chronic pain is associated with higher comorbidities and co-occurrence of substance misuse and substance use disorder (SUD).[7]

Women, particularly young adult women, have become one of the fastest-growing populations with SUD in the US.[8] According to a Substance Abuse and Mental Health Service Administration 2020 report, 17.2 million American women suffered from SUD and 9.5 million women had both SUD and mental illness.[8] Among women with SUD, 7.4 million struggled with illicit drugs, 12.2 million struggled with alcohol use, and 2.5 million struggled with both illicit drugs and alcohol use.[8]

Aside from high rates of mental health comorbidity, women with SUD face various other challenges including a high risk of domestic violence, pregnancy, lack of childcare, economic disadvantage, and social stigma.[8] As an example, college-age women who occasionally drink heavily are at increased risk for assaults and unplanned, unsafe sex.[9] Women veterans with SUD face high rates of trauma, military sexual trauma,

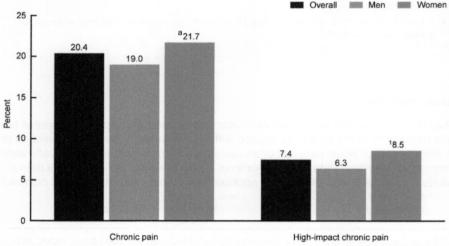

Fig. 1. Percentage of adults aged 18 and over with chronic pain and high-impact chronic pain in the past 3 months, overall and by sex United States, 2019. [a]Significantly different from men ($P<.05$). Notes: Chronic pain is based on responses of "most days" or "every day" to the survey question, "In the past 3 months, how often did you have pain? Would you say never, some days, most days, or every day?" High-impact chronic pain is defined as adults who have chronic pain and who responded, "most days" or "every day" to the survey question, "Over the past 3 months, how often did your pain limit your life or work activities? Would you say never, some days, most days, or every day?" Estimates are based on household interviews of a sample of the civilian noninstitutuinalized population. Access data table for Figure 1 at: http://www.cdc.gov/nchs/data/databriefs/db390-tables-508.pdf#1. (*Data from* National Center for Health Statistics, National Health Interview Survey, 2019.)

higher risk of suicidal behaviors, and social instability.[10] The role of trauma and abuse in women with SUD is not commonly addressed in treatment programs, as most SUD programs are designed for men.[9,10] All these complex factors make it more challenging to manage pain for women with SUD.

Purpose

The purpose of this article is to facilitate a discussion of pain management considerations with practical implications for women with a SUD using the nursing process. The nursing process is incorporated to utilize a systematic framework in women with a SUD. Originally introduced in 1958, the nursing process spans 5 sequential steps: (1) assessment, (2) diagnosis, (3) planning, (4) implementation, and (5) evaluation as a systematic guide to patient-centered care.[11]

BACKGROUND

Substance abuse and substance dependence comprise SUD, using diagnostic criteria derived from DSM-5-TR (outlined in **Table 1**) Alcohol, tobacco, and opioid use disorders are examples of SUDs; however, they may coexist. Beyond general considerations related to a SUD, understanding its intersection with gender-specific factors and pain management is crucial for comprehensive research and targeted interventions. Although the onset of SUD has been historically higher in men, its prevalence is rising for both men and women. The gender gap of SUD is quickly closing amid sociocultural changes for women, such as increased workforce presence and limited access to childcare.[13] Researchers have identified that women face unique challenges with substance use that impact pain management strategies, including genetic, neurohormonal, metabolic, and cultural differences.[13,14] These factors underscore distinctive patterns and outcomes when women are compared to men.

Table 1 DSM-5-TR criteria for substance use disorder	
Criteria	**Description**
Impaired Control	• Taking the substance in larger amounts or over a longer period than was intended. • Wanting to cut down or stop using the substance but being unsuccessful in doing so.
Social Impairment	• Spending a great deal of time getting, using, or recovering from the effects of the substance. • Craving or a strong desire to use the substance. • Failing to fulfill major role obligations at work, school, or home due to substance use.
Risky Use	• Continuing to use the substance despite knowledge of a persistent or recurrent physical or psychological problem that is likely to have been caused or exacerbated by the substance.
Pharmacologic Criteria	• Tolerance: The need for increased amounts of the substance to achieve the desired effect, or a diminished effect with continued use of the same amount. • Withdrawal: The characteristic withdrawal syndrome for the substance, or the use of the substance to relieve or avoid withdrawal symptoms.

At least 2 of the aforementioned criteria must be met within a 12-month period. Severity is determined by the number of symptoms present (mild = 2–3, moderate = 4–5, severe = 6 or more).[12]

DISCUSSION
Diagnosis

When addressing substance use, it is crucial to highlight their significance due their influence on clinical presentation, treatment options, and patient outcomes. Chronic pain is more prevalent among women than men and is a common factor underlying SUD across various healthcare environments.[15,16] As chronic pain diagnoses are greater in women, it is important to note that pain compounds the risk of fatal consequences related to overdose.[15,17] In a recent retrospective review of SUD and chronic non-cancer pain prevalence, the overwhelming majority of patients with SUD had chronic pain, with the most common types involving use of opioids (74.7%), followed by sedatives (72.3%), and cannabis (64.3%).[17] Increased odds for opioid overdose in alcohol and non-opioid use disorders were also reported in those with non-cancer pain.[17] Cannabis use disorder, especially, has been rising among patients with chronic pain in recent years.[18] Traditionally, there were societal perceptions that women had lower rates of substance use compared to men. However, contemporary trends indicate a shift, with increasing acknowledgment of substance use among women. This change is influenced by various factors, including positive trends in workforce participation and improved access to reproductive healthcare.[13]

Contributing Factors to Polysubstance Use in Women

Substance use characteristics are highly dependent on the type of drug, dose, history of drug exposure, environment, and hormonal involvement. Differences in the interplay of pharmacodynamics and pharmacokinetics are additional considerations. One factor is volume of distribution, a theoretic, pharmacokinetic measure referring to the apparent space in the body available to contain a drug. Women have a lower volume of distribution, and therefore exhibit a lower capacity for drug distribution in the body, which results in the drug being confined to the plasma. Thus, women are at higher risk of fatal opioid overdose than men.[9] Additional factors include body weight and metabolism. Women have lower total body weight in comparison to men and metabolize alcohol differently than men, with lower levels of alcohol dehydrogenase on average.[13]

Neurohormonal considerations unique to women also influence both the initial and long-term effects of substances, aside from any future ability to treat related SUD.[13] Researchers have disputed the role of menstrual cycles in drug selection and consumption practices, with more positive effects of substances reported among women in the luteal phase.[13] Studies of exogenous hormone administration lend further evidence to this population. For example, progesterone supplementation has abruptly reduced drug cravings.[13,19] Estrogen interacts differently with alcohol and makes women more prone to develop alcoholic liver disease with faster progression compared to men.[9] Menopause, during which progesterone and estrogen levels decline, leads to masking signs that may adversely affect chronic pain symptoms. Subsequently, mitigation is often sought through polypharmacy.[15] In a study among nearly 105,000 midlife women veterans with chronic pain, menopausal symptoms correlated with providers prescribing risky long-term opioids, which is especially concerning for developing a pain management plan of care.[15]

The courses of SUD, treatment, and pain management are different between the 2 sexes. For example, women initiate substance use later in life than men.[13] Their first use, however, is more likely to be triggered by a traumatic event, such as domestic violence or emotional disturbances.[13] Their patterned trend often follows a more rapid acceleration from first use to problematic use that may impel treatment-seeking.[13] This escalated comportment, which can occur even with minimal substance use, has been regarded as the "telescoping effect," and is especially notable with alcohol, cocaine, and opioid use.[13] Such a rapid progression in women is concomitant with increased cravings, difficulties in treatment, and a heightened likelihood of relapse, further emphasizing the need for gender-specific sensitive approaches and intervention strategies.[14]

Emotional and mental health problems among women are especially concerning. The 2020 National Survey on Drug Use and Health reveals that approximately 9.5 million women, comprising 7.3% of the female population, grapple with the simultaneous challenges of mental illness and SUD.[8] Chronic pain and coexisting rates of mental health diagnoses, such as anxiety and depression, in women lead to a greater likelihood of using substances as a coping mechanism.[13,17] This dual burden underscores the intricate interplay between mental health and substance use among women and emphasizes the necessity for integrated and gender-specific healthcare strategies.

Women with SUD are more likely to seek but underutilize treatment because of historic precedents surrounding stigmatization, childcare issues, and lack of family support. Psychiatric diagnoses compound treatment-seeking likelihood and ability.[13] Women tend to be undertreated, reflecting that their unique needs with differences in pain manifestation and coping patterns are poorly understood.[17] In a cross-sectional study by Escorial and colleagues,[20] women with diagnoses of SUD were more likely than men to present in the emergency department, but also subsequently more likely to be prescribed psychotropic medications. With regard to opioids in the Escorial and colleagues study, women were apt to be prescribed double the modified morphine milligram equivalent of men.[20] Additional research suggests that menopausal women with chronic pain specifically have higher rates of receiving opioids and are prescribed higher doses for a longer duration, co-prescribed with central nervous system depressants.[15,16,21,22] These outcomes likely reflect poor provider understanding of complex pain phenomena and SUD in women.

The continuous high levels of opioid analgesic misuse, consistently around 3.5%, highlight a significant issue in modern healthcare.[8] The primary sources for this misuse are frequently identified as friends or relatives and, notably, one's own prescription.[8] This pattern of misuse raises critical questions about the accessibility and control of prescription medications, necessitating targeted efforts to address the roots of the issue.

Women's polysubstance self-medication practices extend beyond prescription analgesics, encompassing a diverse array of substances. Notably, cannabis is the most commonly used illicit drug, with 16% or approximately 22.9 million women reporting use in the past year.[8] With cannabis, lower doses of delta-9 tetrahydrocannabinol, its main psychoactive substance, lead to abuse potential in women when compared to men.[13,23] Women also respond differently in cannabis use, such as reasons to initiate cannabis use, triggers, response to treatment, and vulnerability to relapse.[9] Contrary to medical advice, there is a rising incidence of women using cannabis (marijuana) during pregnancy. Marijuana has been the most commonly used illicit drug among American young adult women and pregnant women, with approximately 2.8% of pregnant women using it daily or almost daily in the last year.[8,24] SUD during pregnancy can put a developing fetus at significant risk; children who are exposed to drugs prenatally are more likely to develop health or mental health problems and develop SUD in the future.[9] **Fig. 2** denotes substance use patterns among pregnant women in the past month, according to a recent Substance Abuse and Mental Health Services Administration survey.[8]

Women of childbearing age present important issues for thoughtful prescription management and pain control. Opioid use disorder among pregnant women has

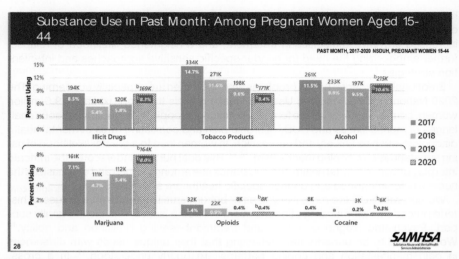

Fig. 2. Substance use in the past month: among pregnant women aged 15-44. [a]Estimate not shown due to low precision. Tobacco products are defined as cigarettes, smokeless tobacco, cigars, and pipe tobacco. [b]Estimates on the 2020 bars are italicized to indicate caution should be used when comparing estimates between 2020 and prior years because of methodological changes for 2020. Due to these changes, significance testing between 2020 and prior years was not performed. 2020 National Survey on Drug Use and Health: Women Substance Abuse and Mental Health Services Administration U.S. Department of Health and Human Services, July 2022. Inclusion of SAMHSA content does not constitute or imply endorsement or recommendation by the Substance Abuse and Mental Health Services Administration, the U.S. Department of Health and Human Services, or the U.S. Government.

quadrupled over a recent 15-year period.[25] Appropriate screening and referral for services, including medication-assisted therapies, are essential maternal health practices. Illicit substance use exposures are on a state-by-state basis as not only adverse maternal but also adverse neonatal outcomes, including preterm labor, abstinence syndrome, and even death, have been linked to opioid exposure.[25]

PLANNING
Management of Plan

In the comprehensive care of pregnant women with a history of opioid use disorder, a meticulous approach to medical and obstetric history is paramount. A thorough assessment provides crucial insights into the context of pain and potential complications. Moreover, it is essential to have a comprehension of the medications approved by the Food and Drug Administration (FDA) for the treatment of opioid use disorder. Refer to **Table 2** for details.

Simultaneously, a rigorous pain assessment, considering the nature, intensity, and duration of pain, should guide the most appropriate interventions.[27] Collaboration within an interdisciplinary team is essential, involving close cooperation with the obstetrician/gynecologist to safeguard both maternal and fetal well-being. The engagement of an addiction specialist is who can oversee buprenorphine therapy and address SUD issues is critical.[28] The management of buprenorphine involves careful prescribing and monitoring, with regular assessments for adherence and signs of misuse. Dose adjustments are made based on pain severity and individual response, and mindful of the potential for respiratory depression.

Table 2
Medications for opioid use disorder used in substance use disorder and consideration for pregnancy

Medication	MOA	Consideration for Pregnancy
Methadone[26,a]	Full mu opioid receptor agonist	Regular assessment of maternal and fetal: Crosses the placenta safer than illicit drugs; adjust doses based on maternal response and fetal well-being; stabilizes cravings and withdrawal
Buprenorphine[26,a]	Partial mu-opioid receptor agonist; Kappa receptor antagonist	Preferred over methadone due to a potentially lower risk of neonatal withdrawal;ceiling effect reduces overdose risk; adjust dosage based on maternal response and fetal well-being.
Naltrexone[26,a]	Mu receptor antagonist	Potential for decreased neonatal withdrawal symptoms; adjust dosage based on maternal response and fetal well-being

[a] The choice of medication should be based on individual patient factors, including the severity of addiction, previous treatment history, and the overall health of the mother and fetus. Consultation with an addiction specialist and obstetrician is crucial for creating a safe and effective treatment plan.

Non-pharmacologic interventions, such as physical therapy for musculoskeletal concerns and psychologic support through counseling or cognitive-behavioral therapy, complement pharmacotherapy interventions (**Table 3**).[29,30] Regular monitoring and follow-up focus on both fetal and maternal health, ensuring the well-being of the developing fetus and addressing potential complications associated with substance use. Patient education involves a comprehensive discussion of the risks and benefits of buprenorphine use during pregnancy, emphasizing the integration of pain management and addiction treatment. Developing a birth plan that considers pain management options during labor and delivery enhances patient-centered care.[27,28,31]

Social determents of health
Addressing social determinants of health (SDOH), such as treatment barriers and access to medication for opioid use disorder and retention, is integral to the care plan.[27] Collaboration with social workers and community resources can provide additional support and resources, fostering a holistic approach. Postpartum planning includes a smooth transition to postpartum care, maintaining ongoing pain management and addiction treatment as needed. Ultimately, achieving a balance in the complexities of pain management with buprenorphine during pregnancy necessitates a patient-centered, interdisciplinary approach. Regular communication among healthcare providers and close monitoring of both maternal and fetal well-being are foundational elements of a successful pain management plan for pregnant women with a history of opioid use disorder.[32]

Multimodal approach. Effective pain management during pregnancy necessitates a comprehensive and multimodal strategy that prioritizes both maternal well-being and the safety of the developing fetus. This approach integrates various interventions to address different facets of pain and enhance overall health.[3] A meticulous assessment by healthcare providers includes evaluating the type, location, and intensity of pain to identify potential underlying causes such as musculoskeletal or neuropathic issues.[26,33]

Table 3
Nonpharmacologic treatment options

Behavioral Therapy Models[29,30]	Focus	Considerations
Cognitive Behavioral Therapy (CBT)	• Identify behavior and response to emotions • Develop coping strategies	• Effective for varying SUDs • Comorbid conditions
Motivational Interviewing (MI)	• Address ambivalence • Build confidence and self-efficacy • Desire for change	• Utilized as brief intervention • Consideration for other supportive models
12-Step Facilitation Therapy	• 12-step peer support models	• Alcoholics Anonymous • Narcotics Anonymous • Motivation • Time
Individual (Interpersonal Therapy)	• Identify areas of focus generated from woman	• Strength-based
Family Therapy/Couple Therapy	• Enhance support • Identify contingency management • Reduce negative impact on the family	• Varying models available • Family training • Reinforcement approach

Non-pharmacologic interventions are a crucial component of care, incorporating physical therapy to address musculoskeletal concerns, safe exercise routines to improve flexibility and circulation, and therapeutic massage and stretching exercises to alleviate muscle tension. Psychologic support, including counseling, cognitive-behavioral therapy, mindfulness, and relaxation techniques help manage emotional aspects of pain, anxiety, and stress. Pharmacologic options like acetaminophen are considered safe for mild to moderate pain relief during pregnancy, while opioids are cautiously used for short durations if the benefits outweigh the risks, with close monitoring for potential adverse effects. Local treatments such as topical analgesics and heat or cold therapy, along with supportive devices like maternity belts and pillows, offer localized relief.

Patient education on proper body mechanics, posture, and nutritional habits further complements the multimodal approach. Regular follow-ups enable healthcare providers to assess the plan's effectiveness and make individualized adjustments based on the patient's response, changing pain patterns, and gestational development. A collaborative interprofessional effort among nursing, obstetricians, pain specialists, physical therapists, and mental health professionals ensures a responsive and tailored pain management plan that aligns with the unique needs of each pregnant woman. Regular communication optimizes relief while minimizing potential risks to both mother and fetus.[34]

IMPLEMENTATION

Evidence-based practice, practice-setting protocols, and national guidelines and legislation should guide the selection of treatment modalities. Despite the ongoing opioid crisis, significant progress has been made,[35] including increased federal funding for research and efforts to sustain an integrated model of delivery of treatment services to individuals with SUDs.[36] The 2023 Consolidated Appropriations Act (CAA) reflects these changes by revoking the previous requirements for the X-waiver (Comprehensive Addiction and Recovery Act of 2016).[37,38] Additionally, this new legislation expands the ability for providers with DEA registration to prescribe buprenorphine (as per the Substance Use-Disorder Prevention that Promotes Opioid Recovery and Treatment for Patients and Communities Act, 2018).[39] Advanced practice nurses wishing to utilize the provisions of the CAA are still required to complete a minimum of 8 h of training focused on the management and treatment of individuals with SUDs. This content should include the current FDA approved treatment options for SUD. The implementation of any treatment plan should begin with careful screening to assess the severity of both pain and substance use. Considering the subjective and complex nature of pain, the individual should guide treatment implementation. The use of Screening, Brief Intervention, and Referral to Treatment has been widely successful in persons with SUDs and can be utilized as a pathway to implementing treatment.[40]

EVALUATION

The evaluation of treatment requires a stepwise evaluation process and should include concepts like short and long-term goals, reduction in severity of symptoms, engagement in treatment, and recovery. The evaluation process should also consider the individual's ability to fulfill normal daily activities with symptom relief and the ability to thrive in their roles.

Case Study

Terry, a 29-year-old woman, presents a complex case of chronic pain management and a long history of SUD. She was diagnosed with fibromyalgia in her twenties and

Table 4
Treatment management guide utilizing the nursing process

Nursing Process	Priority Considerations	Treatment Planning Considerations
Assessment	Medical History	• Fibromyalgia diagnosis • Previous opioid dependence and treatment • Previous diagnosis: anxiety, depression
	Social History	• Limited support system • Employment-related stressors
	Treatment Planning	• Medications for Opioid use Disorder (MOUD) • Buprenorphine initiated to address opioid dependence while minimizing the risk of relapse • Interdisciplinary team: Collaboration with a pain management specialist, addiction psychiatrist, and physical therapist • Cognitive Behavioral Therapy (CBT) • Targeting pain-related anxiety and depressive symptoms • Developing coping strategies for pain flare-ups • Physical therapy and exercise
	Confounding Factors	• Stigma and social isolation • Loss workdays • Expense of multi-treatment modalities
Diagnosis	Comorbid Associations Mental Health Physical Health	• Utilize DSM-5-TR framework • Utilize ICD-10-CM • Prioritize symptom management
Planning	Desired Outcomes	• Prioritize • Person-centered care • Collaborative approach Involvement of woman and family as necessary
Implementation	Resources Consistency SDOH	• Team approach (treatment team) • Identify strength-based strategies • SMART goals
Evaluation	Stepwise Timeline	• Improved pain management • Successful adherence to MOUD, reducing the risk of relapse • Regular attendance in support groups • Enhanced quality of life • Improved mood and overall mental well-being • Re-engagement in social activities

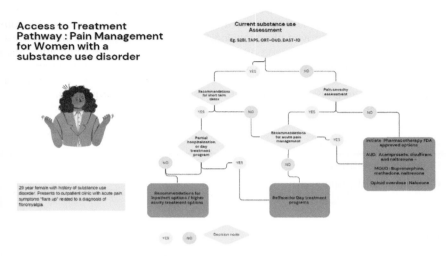

Fig. 3. Decision-making pathway for pain and SUD management. AUD, alcohol use disorder; DAST-10, drug abuse screen test; FDA, U.S. Food and Drug Administration; MOUD, medications for opioid use disorder; ORT-OUD, opioid risk tool–OUD; S2BI, screening to brief intervention; TAPS, tobacco, alcohol, prescription medication, and other substance use.

has struggled with opioid dependence related to that diagnosis. Over the years, she has sought relief through various medications, including opioids, which led to the diagnosis of SUD. Recognizing the need for a holistic approach, Terry is now committed to addressing both her chronic pain and SUD. Utilizing the nursing process, treatment planning considerations can be guided by priority as identified through a shared-decision lens (**Table 4**).

Terry's case highlights the importance of an integrative and personalized approach to pain management for women with SUD. The collaboration of various healthcare professionals, combined with a focus on holistic interventions, has the potential to improve both pain outcomes and the overall well-being of individuals facing this complex dual challenge. Although multi-modal options for treatment are available for this population, there remains a need for ongoing research and development of tailored interventions for young women with SUD. Positive outcomes also require deliberate collaboration of all providers involved with Terry's treatment and Terry's participation in the decision-making process. Utilizing the availability of treatment options, empowering the woman to choose based on their needs, and a shared decision-making process between patient and provider can promote sustained engagement and improved treatment outcomes (**Fig. 3**).[41,42]

SUMMARY

The intricate relationship between chronic pain and SUD in women is challenging due to multifaceted factors, including mental health, trauma, and societal challenges. Utilizing the nursing process, this article provides a systematic approach to pain management for women with polysubstance use, emphasizing 5 sequential steps: assessment, diagnosis, planning, implementation, and evaluation. Women, particularly young adults, are identified as a rapidly increasing population affected by SUD in the US.[8] This population yields special considerations for gender-specific challenges, such as domestic violence, pregnancy, childcare, and social stigma, further influencing pain management strategies. Emphasis should be placed on a comprehensive approach to pain management, including FDA-approved pharmacologic and non-pharmacologic interventions, interprofessional collaboration, and addressing SDOH. Personalized and integrative approaches to pain management for women with SUD are important. This article advocates for ongoing research, the development of tailored interventions, and empowering women through shared decision-making for improved treatment outcomes.

CLINICS CARE POINTS

- Complex interrelationship.
- Systematic nursing approach.
- Gender-specific challenges.
- Comprehensive pain management.
- A personalized and integrative care.

DISCLOSURES

The authors have nothing to disclose.

REFERENCES

1. Amini M, Pourshahbaz A, Mohammadkhani P, et al. The relationship between five-factor model and diagnostic and statistical manual of mental disorder-fifth edition personality traits on patients with antisocial personality disorder. J Res Med Sci 2015;20(5):470–6.
2. Nahin RL, Sayer B, Stussman BJ, et al. Eighteen-year trends in the prevalence of, and health care use for, noncancer pain in the United States: data from the Medical Expenditure Panel Survey. J Pain 2019;20(7):796–809.
3. Treede RD. The International Association for the Study of Pain definition of pain: as valid in 2018 as in 1979, but in need of regularly updated footnotes. Pain Rep 2018;3(2):e643.
4. Zelaya CE, Dahlhamer JM, Lucas JW, et al. Chronic pain and high-impact chronic pain among U.S. adults, 2019. NCHS Data Brief 2020;390:1–8.
5. Yong RJ, Mullins PM, Bhattacharyya N. Prevalence of chronic pain among adults in the United States. Pain 2022;163(2):e328–32.
6. Center for Disease Control and Prevention. National center for health Statistics. National Health Interview Survey 2021. Available at: https://www.cdc.gov/nchs/nhis/2019nhis.htm. Accessed January 24, 2024.
7. Ilgen MA, Bohnert ASB, Chermack S, et al. A randomized trial of a pain management intervention for adults receiving substance use disorder treatment. Addiction 2016;111(8):1385–93.
8. Substance Abuse and Mental Health Services Administration, 2020 national survey on drug use and health: women, 2022, Center for Behavioral Health Statistics and Quality, Substance Abuse and Mental Health Services Administration; Rockville, MD. Available at: https://www.samhsa.gov/data/report/2020-nsduh-women. (Accessed 20 April 2024).
9. Ait-Daoud N, Blevins D, Khanna S, et al. Women and addiction. Psychiatric Clin North Am 2017;40(2):285–97.

10. Hoggatt KJ, Lehavot K, Krenek M, et al. Prevalence of substance misuse among US veterans in the general population. Am J Addict 2017;26(4):357–65.
11. Toney-Butler TJ, Thayer JM. Nursing process. In: StatPearls. StatPearls Publishing; 2023. Available at: http://www.ncbi.nlm.nih.gov/books/NBK499937/. Accessed January 7, 2024.
12. American Psychiatric Association. Diagnostic and statistical manual of mental disorders. 5th, text revision edition. Washington, DC: American Psychiatric Publishing; 2022.
13. McHugh RK, Votaw VR, Sugarman DE, et al. Sex and gender differences in substance use disorders. Clin Psychol Rev 2018;66:12–23.
14. National Institute on Drug Abuse. Substance use in women research report. 2020. Available at: https://nida.nih.gov/publications/drugfacts/substance-use-in-women. Accessed November 13, 2023.
15. Gibson CJ, Li Y, Huang AJ, et al. Menopausal symptoms and higher risk opioid prescribing in a national sample of women veterans with chronic pain. J Gen Intern Med 2019;34:2159–66.
16. Higgins DM, Kerns RD, Brandt CA, et al. Persistent pain and comorbidity among operation enduring freedom/operation Iraqi freedom/operation new dawn veterans. Pain Med 2014;15(5):782–90.
17. John WS, Wu LT. Chronic non-cancer pain among adults with substance use disorders: prevalence, characteristics, and association with opioid overdose and healthcare utilization. Drug Alcohol Depend 2020;209:107902.
18. Reece AS, Hulse GK. Quadruple convergence – rising cannabis prevalence, intensity, concentration and use disorder treatment. Lancet Reg Health Eur 2021. https://doi.org/10.1016/j.lanepe.2021.100245.
19. Milivojevic V, Fox HC, Sofuoglu M, et al. Effects of progesterone stimulated allopregnanolone on craving and stress response in cocaine dependent men and women. Psychoneuroendocrinology 2016;65:44–53.
20. Escorial M, Muriel J, Margarit C, et al. Sex-differences in pain and opioid use disorder management: a cross-sectional real-world study. Biomedicines 2022;10(9):2302.
21. Mosher HJ, Krebs EE, Carrel M, et al. Trends in prevalent and incident opioid receipt: an observational study in Veterans Health Administration 2004–2012. J Gen Intern Med 2015;30(5):597–604.
22. Kroll-Desrosiers AR, Skanderson M, Bastian LA, et al. Receipt of prescription opioids in a national sample of pregnant veterans receiving Veterans Health Administration care. Wom Health Issues 2016;26(2):240–6.
23. Fogel JS, Kelly TH, Westgate PM, et al. Sex differences in the subjective effects of oral Δ9-THC in cannabis users. Pharmacol Biochem Behav 2017;152:44–51.
24. Qato DM, Zhang C, Gandhi AB, et al. Co-use of alcohol, tobacco, and licit and illicit controlled substances among pregnant and non-pregnant women in the United States: findings from 2006 to 2014 National Survey on Drug Use and Health (NSDUH) data. Drug Alcohol Depend 2020;206:107729.
25. Haight SC, Ko JY, Tong VT, et al. Opioid use disorder documented at delivery hospitalization — United States, 1999–2014. MMWR Morb Mortal Wkly Rep 2018;67(31):845–9.
26. National Institute on Drug Abuse. How effective are medications to treat opioid use disorder?. 2021. Available at: https://nida.nih.gov/publications/research-reports/medications-to-treat-opioid-addiction/efficacy-medications-opioid-use-disorder. Accessed January 24, 2024.
27. Harrison TK, Kornfeld H, Aggarwal AK, et al. Perioperative considerations for the patient with opioid use disorder on buprenorphine, methadone, or naltrexone

maintenance therapy. Anesthesiol Clin 2018;36(3):345–59. https://doi.org/10.1016/j.anclin.2018.04.002.

28. Shulman M, Wai JM, Nunes EV. Buprenorphine treatment for opioid use disorder: an overview. CNS Drugs 2019;33(6):567–80. https://doi.org/10.1007/s40263-019-00637-z.

29. Quality Forum National. Behavioral health 2016-2017 final report. 2017. Available at: https://www.qualityforum.org/Publications/2017/08/Behavioral_Health_2016-2017_Final_Report.aspx. Accessed January 24, 2024.

30. Marcovitz DE, McHugh KR, Roos C, et al. Overlapping mechanisms of recovery between professional psychotherapies and Alcoholics Anonymous. J Addict Med 2020;14(5):367–75.

31. U.S. Department of Health & Human Services. Overdose prevention strategy. 2021. Available at: https://www.hhs.gov/overdose-prevention/. Accessed January 24, 2024.

32. Radic M, Parlier-Ahmad AB, Wills B, et al. Social determinants of health and emergency department utilization among adults receiving buprenorphine for opioid use disorder. Drug Alcohol Depend Rep 2022;3:100062 [published correction appears in Drug Alcohol Depend Rep. 2022 Dec;5].

33. Kohan L, Potru S, Barreveld AM, et al. Buprenorphine management in the perioperative period: educational review and recommendations from a multisociety expert panel. Reg Anesth Pain Med 2021;46(10):840–59.

34. Krashin D, Murnova N, Ballantyne J. Multidisciplinary management of acute and chronic pain in the presence of substance use disorder (SUD). In: el-Guebaly N, Carrà G, Galanter M, editors. Textbook of addiction treatment: international perspectives. 2nd edition. Cham, Switzerland: Springer; 2021. p. 535–46.

35. Centers for Disease Control and Prevention. Waves of the opioid epidemic. 2023. Available at: https://www.cdc.gov/opioids/basics/epidemic.html. Accessed January 24, 2024.

36. Substance use prevention, treatment, and recovery services block grant Act of 2022, H.R.7235, 117th cong. (2021-2022). Congress.gov. 2022. Available at: https://www.congress.gov/bill/117th-congress/house-bill/7235. Accessed January 29, 2024.

37. Consolidations Appropriations Act of 2023. (2023). P.L. 117-328. Available at: https://www.policymed.com/wp-content/uploads/2023/01/CME-DEA-Omnibus-Bill-2023-Clean-Version-R. Accessed January 28, 2024.

38. Comprehensive addiction and recovery Act of 2016: P.L. 114-198, Available at: https://www.congress.gov/114/plaws/publ198/PLAW-114publ198.pdf, (Accessed 30 August 2024), 2016.

39. Substance use-disorder prevention that promotes opioid recovery and treatment for patients and Communities Act or the SUPPORT for patients and Communities Act: P.L. 115-271. 2018. Available at: https://www.congress.gov/bill/115th-congress/house-bill/6. Accessed January 24, 2024.

40. Substance Abuse and Mental Health Services Administration. SBIRT: screening, brief intervention, and referral to treatment. 2022. Available at: https://www.samhsa.gov/sbirt. Accessed January 28, 2024.

41. Marshall T, Hancock M, Kinnard EN, et al. Treatment options and shared decision-making in the treatment of opioid use disorder: a scoping review. J Subst Abuse Treat 2022;135:108646. https://doi.org/10.1016/j.jsat.2021.108646.

42. US Food and Drug Administration (FDA). Information about medication-assisted treatment (MAT). 2023. Available at: https://www.fda.gov/drugs/information-drug-class/information-about-medication-assisted-treatment-mat. Accessed January 24, 2024.

Caring for Transgender Patients

Shivon Latice Daniels, MSN, APRN, FNP-C[a],*,
Jacquetta Woods Melvin, MPH, PA-C[b],
Quinnette Jones, MSW, MHS, PA-C[b]

KEYWORDS

- Transgender • Feminizing • Masculinizing • Gender diversity • Gender identity

KEY POINTS

- Transgender-diverse patients experience significant health disparities.
- Inclusive care is important with caring for transgender-diverse patients.
- Understanding the health maintenance needs of transgender-diverse patients is essential.
- Transgender-diverse patients have various options of gender-affirming treatments that are important for health care providers to understand when caring for transgender patients.

INTRODUCTION

The number of people who openly identify as transgender or gender diverse (TGD) is increasing and nurses must be prepared to provide inclusive care to all patients across clinical settings.[1] People who are TGD have a gender identity that differs from their sex assigned at birth. TGD people may identify as transgender women/transfeminine, transgender men/transmasculine, nonbinary/genderqueer, agender,[2] or as another identity not listed (**Table 1**). People who are transgender currently represent 0.6% of the United States population; however among Millennials (born 1981–1996) and Generation Z (born 1997–2004), they represent 1.0% and 1.9% of the populations, respectively.[1] Given these demographic shifts, nurses can expect to see increased numbers of patients who are TGD and need to be appropriately prepared to address their health needs.

TGD patients experience significant health disparities including stigmatization and discrimination in health care settings.[5] Among TGD people, 25% have been refused

[a] Duke Heath Integrative Practice, Department of Medicine, Division of Endocrinology, Metabolism, and Nutrition, DUMC 3021 Durham, NC 27710, USA; [b] Department of Family Medicine & Community Health, Division of PA Studies, Duke University, 800 South Duke Street, Durham, NC 27710, USA
* Corresponding author.
E-mail address: Shivon.Daniels@duke.edu

Nurs Clin N Am 59 (2024) 625–635
https://doi.org/10.1016/j.cnur.2024.07.015   **nursing.theclinics.com**

Table 1
Gender-related definitions & terminology[3,4]

Term	Definition	Examples[a]
Sex	Physical characteristics based on anatomic, genetic, and biological factors	Female, Male, Intersex
Gender	Characteristics and roles based on social and cultural norms and are socially constructed	Man, woman, girl, boy, transgender woman, transgender man, transfeminine, transmasculine, nonbinary, genderqueer, gender fluid, agender
Gender Identity	A person's inner sense of their gender	
Gender Diversity	Term that describes the spectrum of gender identities and expressions that may or may not align with assigned sex	
		Nonbinary — A term used to describe gender identity that does not conform to traditional binary gender identities. May include a combination of binary identities.
		Genderqueer — Term that describes gender identities that do not adhere to the traditional binary identities
		Agender — Term used when a person does not identify using gender
		Transgender — See below
Transgender Identity	A person's identity that differs from their sex assigned at birth	Transgender woman — A person who was assigned male sex at birth and identifies as a woman
		Transfeminine — Term to describe a person who was assigned male at birth and identifies more with femininity than masculinity.
		Transgender man — A person who was assigned female at birth and identifies as a man
		Transmasculine — Term to describe a person who was assigned female at birth and identifies more with masculinity than femininity

[a] Examples are not an exhaustive list of all identities within a group.

medical care related to their gender identity and over one-third have had to teach their health care team about their gender diversity in order to receive appropriate care.[6] These experiences cause TGD patients to delay or avoid care[6] and can lead to poor physical and mental health outcomes. People who are TGD have higher rates of depression, anxiety, suicide attempts, smoking, and substance use than the general population.[7] They are less likely to have a regular health care provider[8] and to be up to date on screenings such as those for cervical cancer, breast cancer, and prostate cancer.[9]

Nurses working in traditional "women's health" settings such as obstetrics and gynecology, breast and gynecologic specialties, or primary care may see patients across the gender spectrum including those who are transfeminine, transmasculine, or nonbinary. A patient who was assigned female at birth and identifies as a transgender man may present for a gender-affirming gynecologic examination or for obstetric care in one of these clinical settings. Nonbinary and transfeminine patients may have traditional "women's health" needs such as breast cancer screenings in addition to traditionally considered "men's health" needs based on their anatomy. The authors suggest against use of binary terms for health care, such as men's or women's health, which are not inclusive of all genders. As central members of the health care team, nurses are well-positioned to support an inclusive culture for gender-diverse patients across specialties. This article aims to provide the appropriate terminology, an overview of gender-affirming treatments, and recommendations for nurses in the care of patients who are gender diverse.

LANGUAGE AND TERMINOLOGY

Inclusive care requires understanding the terminology and appropriately using terms, names, and pronouns. See **Table 1** for definitions of commonly used terminology. Diagnoses that may be used when caring for patients who are TGD include gender dysphoria and gender incongruence. Gender dysphoria is a term that was first included in the American Psychiatric Association's Diagnostic and Statistical Manual-5 in in 2013[10] and describes an incongruence between a person's gender identity and their sex assigned at birth.[11] Gender incongruence is a term recognized by the International Classification of Diseases and Related Health Problems, 11th Version of the World Health Organization (ICD-11) which does not imply gender diversity is pathologic.[12] Despite this advantage of the use of gender incongruence, a diagnosis of gender dysphoria is still often necessary in the United States to obtain insurance coverage for gender care.[12]

When caring for people who are TGD, nurses should ensure they use the patient's correct pronouns. If unsure of the patient's pronouns, then it would be appropriate to address the patient by their name.[13] The nurse may share their pronouns and ask the patient what pronouns they use or what they would like to be called. Incorrect pronoun use reinforces the negative experiences of people who are TGD making it even more important for nurses to promote an inclusive space. If a mistake occurs, an apology should be offered to prevent the patient from feeling further stigmatized and victimized within the health care system. See **Table 2** for additional strategies that can be used to promote an inclusive environment.

Gender-Neutral Language

Gender-neutral language is language that includes everyone regardless of their gender identity making it an inclusive way to communicate with all patients. Some patients may not be comfortable with gendered terms such as *breasts* if having breasts

Table 2
Promoting inclusive patient encounters[14-16]

Creating an Inclusive Space	Examples
Ask the patient's preferred name	"What would you like me to call you?" or "What name do you like to go by?"
Share your name and pronouns	"My name is_ and I use she/her pronouns." Wear a pin with your pronouns
Ask what pronouns the patient uses	"What pronouns do you use?" • He/him/his • She/her/hers • They/them/their
Acknowledge when non-inclusive language is used	Apologize if you or others make a mistake with pronouns, name, etc.
Consider the physical environment	Display a non-discrimination statement, know the location of all gender or single stall bathrooms
Use gender-neutral language and/or mirror the patient's language	Use the term chest instead of *breasts or bleeding* instead of *menstrual cycle* if the patient uses these terms

contributes to their gender dysphoria. In such situations, use of gender neutral language such as *chest* may create a more comfortable encounter. In other situations, use of a gendered term such as *mothering* may exclude the experience of another parent when use of the term *parenting* would be more inclusive. An important aspect of using language in patient encounters is to mirror the patient's language when possible. Some patients who are TGD may prefer gendered terms to describe themselves or their anatomy highlighting the importance of understanding the patient's preferences. See **Table 3** for examples of gender neutral terminology.

HEALTH MAINTENANCE FOR TRANSGENDER OR GENDER DIVERSE PEOPLE

A majority of health issues affecting TGD people are no different from those of the remainder of the population, and most medical care sought by transgender patients is unrelated to their gender identity.[20] As with cisgender patients, providers should determine the purpose of the patient's visit and tailor the history and physical to specific patient needs. It is essential for all providers to consider specialized components

Table 3
Examples of gender-neutral language in health care[17-19]

Instead of	Try
Men, Women, Females, Males	Person, People, or Everyone
Mothering/Fathering	Parenting
Pregnant woman	Pregnant Person
Maternity Leave	Parental Leave
Well Woman Examination	Well Person Examination
Breasts/Breastfeeding	Chest/Chest feeding
Menstrual Cycle/Period	Bleeding
Birth Control	Contraception

of a sensitive history and physical examination, and develop a sensitive approach to ensure patient safety and comfort during the health care visit.

For both transfeminine and transmasculine patients, a history should include past medical history and surgical history, an organ inventory, chronic health conditions, medications, social history, family history, substance use, and mental health screening. A physical examination should be completed after providing anticipatory communication and discussing which components of the physical examination will be performed. It is recommended that breast, genital, and rectal examinations are only performed when necessary, and a chaperone should always be offered.[20]

When providing preventative health care, health screenings should be based on the anatomy present rather than the patient's gender identity.[20] In most cases, screening guidelines for transgender patients align with screening guidelines for cisgender patients with the same anatomy. Transfeminine patients over the age of 50 who have used feminizing hormones for at least 5 years should have screening mammography performed every 1 to 2 years.[20,21] Transmasculine patients who have not undergone a hysterectomy should continue to receive cervical cancer screenings.[22] It is important to note that transfeminine patients do retain their prostates even after undergoing gender-affirming surgeries[23] and examination may not be possible by digital rectal examination.[24] There are no current guidelines for prostate screening in transfeminine patients; the World Professional Association for Transgender Health recommends offering the same screenings that are offered to cisgender men.[25] Additionally, Centers for Disease Control and Prevention recommendations for vaccinations in transgender patients do not differ from that of cisgender patients.[20]

GENDER-AFFIRMING TREATMENTS

Medically necessary gender-affirming hormonal therapy (GAHT) can decrease gender dysphoria and improve quality of life.[26,27] GAHT is managed by licensed medical providers and supports alignment of as secondary sex characteristics to align with a person's gender identity. GAHT may be prescribed in different formulations including pills, patches, gels, or injections.[28] Prior to initiating treatment, discussion regarding the patient's goals and expectations in addition to risks and benefits of treatment should be documented.[29] The patient's reproductive health and fertility should be discussed prior to starting treatment. Prior to starting GAHT, a comprehensive medical assessment and baseline laboratory testing is obtained.[27] After starting hormone therapy, patients who are TGD are typically seen at intervals of every 3 months with laboratory monitoring. Visits may become less frequent over time once GAHT doses are stable.[27]

Hormone Treatments

Feminizing

Patients receiving feminizing GAHT may desire full or partial feminization depending on their goals for treatment. Feminizing GAHT treatment focuses on the development of secondary feminine characteristics.[30] TGD patients on feminizing hormone therapy may be taking estrogen alone although it is often used in combination with an anti-androgen medication to help suppress secondary male characteristics.[28] Estrogen is available in different formulations including pills, patches, and injections. Oral estrogen may be taken once or twice daily while transdermal patches are typically placed twice weekly. Injectable estrogen may be taken intramuscularly weekly or every 2 weeks or subcutaneously once weekly.[31,32] Estrogen use may be associated with an increased risk of venous thromboembolism.[28,33] Because transdermal estrogen bypasses metabolism in the liver and may reduce this risk, it may be preferred for patients over the age of forty and in those who smoke.[30]

Anti-androgens are often used along with estrogen because estrogen alone may not be enough to suppress androgens, or male sex hormones such as testosterone. The most commonly used anti-androgen medication is spironolactone. Spironolactone is a potassium-sparing diuretic and is used to treat hypertension and heart failure, and also acts to reduce testosterone levels. Electrolytes may be monitored via routine laboratory studies.[28,34] Evidence is limited on the use of progesterone for feminizing effects; however, it is often used as adjunctive treatment for additional breast development or improving libido, or mood.[29]

Physical changes that occur with feminizing gender-affirming hormone therapy may include breast development, body fat redistribution, softening of the skin, decreased muscle mass, decreased sperm production, decreased sexual desire, and decreased terminal hair growth[28,29] Most patients will start seeing physical changes within the first 3 to 6 months. A decrease in libido or erections may be seen as early as 1 to 3 months.[29] Other effects from GAHT will progress over the course of several years. Breast development is a permanent physical change while other changes may be reversible in the absence of estrogen treatment.

Masculinizing

TGD patients seeking full or partial masculinizing hormones are prescribed testosterone, which is a controlled substance in the United States.[35] Formulations of testosterone include oral, transdermal, and injectable testosterone, which can be taken intramuscularly or subcutaneously.[36] Oral and transdermal testosterone are typically taken once daily while injectable may be used weekly for subcutaneous or every 2 weeks if intramuscular.[32] The physical changes which can be expected with masculinizing hormone therapy include facial and body hair growth, acne and skin oiliness, clitoral enlargement or "bottom growth," deeper voice, increase in libido, increased muscle mass, and body fat redistribution.[27] Physical changes may begin within a few months of initiating treatment and progress of the course of several years.[36] Irreversible changes of testosterone use include facial and body hair growth, deepening of the voice, and clitoral enlargement. Acne, changes in libido, muscle mass, and body fat redistribution are reversible after stopping testosterone therapy. Testosterone therapy often also results in amenorrhea, particularly at higher doses. If menstruation continues and is dysphoric for the patient, a progestin may be prescribed to prevent bleeding. It is important to note that although the patient may experience amenorrhea from testosterone, contraception is needed as pregnancy can still occur.[27] Testosterone treatment can result in changes to a patient's lipids and red blood cell counts which are monitored as part of treatment.[36]

Surgical Interventions

Gender-affirming surgeries are becoming increasingly common in the United States. Among medically treated transgender persons, surveys suggest that approximately half seek transgender-specific surgical procedures.[7] Similar to GAHT, gender-affirming surgical procedures allow closer alignment with a patient's body and gender identity. Gender-affirming surgery consists of many different procedures, including non-breast, non-genital surgeries (ie, facial feminization procedures), "top"(breast) surgeries, and "bottom"(genital) surgeries.[37] For many transgender and gender-diverse patients, gender-affirming surgery is a critical aspect of their overall health and wellness and has a significant impact on their social functioning.[38] For nurses who provide care in perioperative settings, special attention to unique aspects of

TGD perioperative care is essential. For the purpose of this article, only the transfeminine and transmasculine "bottom" procedures are discussed. With the exception of potential need for additional mental health consideration, perioperative considerations for TGD patients who undergo non-genital surgeries are similar to those of cisgender patients.[37]

For both feminizing-affirming and masculinizing-affirming surgical procedures, preoperative care should include infectious disease management, hormone management, bariatric considerations, and reproductive planning.[38] Additionally, mental health is a critical aspect in the preparation for gender-affirming surgery. Some gender-affirming surgeries require preoperative psychological assessments from mental health clinicians that identify any psychiatric diagnoses, evaluate a patient's eligibility for surgery, and confirm capacity for informed consent.

Feminizing

For feminizing surgical interventions, transgender women may undergo vaginoplasty to create a neovagina. Procedures involved in a vaginoplasty include removal of the penis and testes, and creation of the vagina, clitoris, and vulva.[39] Post-operatively, patients are treated with antibiotics while retaining a urinary catheter and vaginal packing in place. Both urinary catheter and vaginal packing are removed at the 1 week follow-up visit. After vaginal packing is removed, patients are advised to douche at least 1 to 2 times per week. This is advised in order to compensate for the lack of an acidic natal pH; thus, preventing bacterial overgrowth and excessive discharge. Patients are also instructed to follow a daily dilator regimen with progressively larger dilators.[37]

Post-operative complications to consider in the first week are similar to those after other major surgeries (ie, venous thromboembolism, urinary tract infection, pulmonary atelectasis, and pneumonia). The patient's symptoms should guide clinical reasoning and diagnostic testing. If the patient still has a urinary catheter, ensure tubing is correctly positioned without clogs or kinks. Specific to the procedure itself are urologic and surgical wound complications, so the pelvic examination is an important part of the physical examination. If the vaginal packing is still in place, a pelvic examination should not be performed.[39]

Masculinizing

For masculinizing surgical interventions, among transgender men, 24% of patients subsequently undergo phalloplasty, or creation of male genital structures, with a staged erection or testicular prostheses implantation.[37] Because these are staged procedures that may span months or years, it is important to understand where the patient is in their process. Skin flaps from the radial forearm and anterolateral thigh are the most common donor sites used to create the neophallus. Post-operatively, patients are discharged with a suprapubic catheter for up to 4 weeks while the neophallus heals. Patients are advised to avoid penetrative intercourse for 3 months.[39] Similar to transfeminine and other major surgeries, postoperative complications in the first week include venous thromboembolism, urinary tract infection, pulmonary atelectasis, and pneumonia, and the patient's suprapubic catheter should be evaluated to ensure correct positioning, and to ensure it is not clogged or has kinks.[39] Additionally, the flap donor site should be assessed for infection or ischemia from arterial or venous occlusion. One week post operatively, complications primarily involve the urinary tract or surgical wound. It's imperative that when evaluating a transmasculine patient for abdominal pain, health care providers remember that they may still have their internal pelvic reproductive organs.[37,39]

It is essential for all health care providers to expand their knowledge of gender-affirming surgery, as TGD patients who undergo gender- affirming procedures may present to a variety of clinical setting for perioperative surgical care. Having a basic understanding of these procedures and their complications may improve, and ensure, optimal care of these patients.

DISCUSSION

The American Nurses Association (ANA), like the majority of major health care associations,[40] opposes restrictions on transgender health care.[41] The ANA published their statement of opposition in 2022 in response to the legislative efforts to restrict access to gender-affirming care in a number of states.[41] Unfortunately, the number of anti-trans legislative efforts has continued to rise since then. At the time of this article, 496 bills had already been introduced in 2024 and 2023 saw 3 times more bills than prior years. Bills affecting TGD youth's ability to participate in sports have been passed in over one-third of states in the United States and legislation restricting their access to gender-affirming care has introduced in record numbers.[42] Bills affecting TGD people's bathroom usage and their ability to update government identification are also growing.[42] These policies negatively impact the mental health and well-being of TGD people by increasing stigmatization, internally and externally, and creating a hostile environment. Increased depression and anxiety have been found in TGD youth in response to these legislative efforts. Policies shape social determinants of health and anti-trans legislation has the potential to worsen the disparities experienced by people who are TGD.[40]

The topic of detransitioning, when a person who is transgender decides to stop or reverse treatments, deserves discussion as it is often raised as a counter-argument to gender-affirming care. Detransitioning, which is sometimes referred to as retransitioning, describes a variety of situations which may include reidentification with sex assigned at birth or maintenance of a transgender identity without continued treatments. It is important to note that detransitioning is not synonymous with regret and not all patients who detransition report regret. Estimates for rates of detransition following hormonal or surgical treatments range from 0% to 9.8%.[43] Despite these low rates, nurses should be prepared to support patients who discontinue treatment by ensuring linkage to appropriate medical, mental health, and social supports.[44]

SUMMARY

Nurses may find themselves caring for patients who are TGD in any clinical setting. With adequate knowledge about the needs of TGD patients and use of inclusive practices, they can support improved health care experiences for these patients. People who are TGD may transition socially, medically, or surgically depending on their treatment goals. Medical transitioning typically involves either estrogen alone or in combination with an anti-androgen medication or testosterone depending on whether it is feminizing or masculinizing. Numerous surgical options for patients who are TGD with nursing needs and recovery times vary depending on the procedure. Health maintenance for patients who are TGD should be based on the anatomy present.

CLINICS CARE POINTS

- Using the patient's correct name, pronouns, gender-neutral language and mirroring patients' language promotes a more inclusive and welcoming environment.

- Preventative health care and routine screenings should be offered based on anatomy present and risks.
- Medically necessary hormone therapy is an effective and safe treatment that improves quality of life for patients who are transgender and gender diverse. It is prescribed by licensed medical providers who monitor laboratory and clinical findings regularly.
- Feminizing hormone therapy typically includes estrogen and an anti-androgen medication. Physical changes that occur with feminizing hormone therapy include breast growth, fat redistribution, decreased muscle mass, softening of the skin, and decreased libido and/or erections.
- Testosterone is the mainstay of masculinizing hormone therapy. Physical changes that occur with masculinizing hormone therapy include clitoral enlargement, body fat redistribution, body and facial hair, deepening of the voice, and increased muscle mass.
- For TGD patients considering surgical procedures, approach conversations and interactions with openness and sensitivity. Many TGD patients find health care interactions overwhelmingly triggering given past experiences.
- The peri-operative period can be a specifically challenging and vulnerable time for TGD patients as they manage navigating the health care system to receive operative care. Additionally, post-operative complications can further exacerbate these challenges. It is important that nurses remain vigilant, ensuring detailed reports and hand-offs occur between care providers throughout different stages in patients care. Overall, thoughtful and inclusive patient care throughout the entirety of the perioperative period is essential to the safe and successful management of TGD patients.

REFERENCES

1. Jones JUS. LGBT Identification Steady at 7.2%. Gallup.com. 2023. Available at: https://news.gallup.com/poll/470708/lgbt-identification-steady.aspx. Accessed June 21, 2023.
2. Transgender and Gender Diverse Persons. 2022. Available at: https://www.cdc.gov/std/treatment-guidelines/trans.htm. Accessed January 22, 2024.
3. Reisner SL, Keuroghlian AS, Potter J. Gender Identity: Terminology, Demographics, and Epidemiology. In: Keuroghlian AS, Potter J, Reisner SL, eds Transgender and Gender Diverse Health Care: The Fenway Guide. McGraw Hill; 2022. Available at: accessmedicine.mhmedical.com/content.aspx?aid=1184175780. Accessed June 21, 2023.
4. Zavaletta V, Allen BJ, Parikh AK. Re-defining gender diversity through an equitable and inclusive lens. Pediatr Radiol 2022;52(9):1743–8.
5. Jaffee KD, Shires DA, Stroumsa D. Discrimination and Delayed Health Care Among Transgender Women and Men: Implications for Improving Medical Education and Health Care Delivery. Med Care 2016;54(11):1010–6.
6. Gruberg S, Mahowald L, Jalpin J. The State of the LGBTQ Community in 2020. Center for American Progress. 2020. Available at: https://www.americanprogress.org/article/state-lgbtq-community-2020/. Accessed January 18, 2024.
7. Safer JD, Coleman E, Feldman J, et al. Barriers to health care for transgender individuals. Curr Opin Endocrinol Diabetes Obes 2016;23(2):168–71.
8. Dawson L, Long M, Published BF. LGBT+ people's health status and access to care - issue brief - 10171. KFF. Published June 30, 2023. Available at: https://www.kff.org/report-section/lgbt-peoples-health-status-and-access-to-care-issue-brief/. Accessed January 18, 2024.
9. Leone AG, Trapani D, Schabath MB, et al. Cancer in transgender and gender-diverse persons: a review. JAMA Oncol 2023;9(4):556–63.

10. Crocq MA. How gender dysphoria and incongruence became medical diagnoses - a historical review. Dialogues Clin Neurosci 2021;23(1):44–51.

11. Patel H, Camacho JM, Salehi N, et al. Journeying through the hurdles of gender-affirming care insurance: a literature analysis. Cureus 2023;15(3):e36849.

12. Gomez I, Ranji U, Salganicoff A, et al. Update on medicaid coverage of gender-affirming health services. KFF. Published October 11, 2022. Available at: https://www.kff.org/womens-health-policy/issue-brief/update-on-medicaid-coverage-of-gender-affirming-health-services/. Accessed March 4, 2024.

13. Jha S, Bouman WP. Introduction to healthcare for transgender and gender-diverse people. Best Pract Res Clin Obstet Gynaecol 2023;87:102299.

14. Cicero EC, Wesp LM. Supporting the health and well-being of transgender students. J Sch Nurs 2017;33(2):95–108.

15. Salazar P. How to Use Inclusive Language in Healthcare. CORP-MSN0 (NLM). Published April 16, 2021. Available at: https://nursinglicensemap.com/blog/how-to-use-inclusive-language-in-healthcare/. Accessed March 4, 2024.

16. Creating an LGBTQ-friendly practice. American Medical Association. Published March 9, 2024. Available at: https://www.ama-assn.org/delivering-care/population-care/creating-lgbtq-friendly-practice. Accessed March 15, 2024.

17. Pronouns Are a Public Health Issue - ProQuest. Available at: https://www.proquest.com/docview/2638091809?parentSessionId=ZHSOnlogEn6woEs9UKIQWrOgaJ6TbSQaQ1wpPdVjVC8%3D&sourcetype=Scholarly%20Journals. Accessed March 4, 2024.

18. The 2 sides of using gender-neutral language in healthcare. J Perinat Neonatal Nurs 2023;37(4):267.

19. Inclusive and Gender-Neutral Language. National Institutes of Health (NIH). Published August 11, 2022. Available at: https://www.nih.gov/nih-style-guide/inclusive-gender-neutral-language. Accessed March 4, 2024.

20. Whitlock BL, Duda ES, Elson MJ, et al. Primary care in transgender persons. Endocrinol Metab Clin North Am 2019;48(2):377–90.

21. Clarke CN, Cortina CS, Fayanju OM, et al. Breast cancer risk and screening in transgender persons: a call for inclusive care. Ann Surg Oncol 2022;29(4):2176–80.

22. Guelbert C. Nursing considerations for transgender men. Nursing (Lond). 2022;52(1):18–22.

23. Nik-Ahd F, Jarjour A, Figueiredo J, et al. Prostate-specific antigen screening in transgender patients. Eur Urol 2023;83(1):48–54.

24. Bertoncelli Tanaka M, Sahota K, Burn J, et al. Prostate cancer in transgender women: what does a urologist need to know? BJU Int 2022;129(1):113–22.

25. Standards of Care - WPATH World Professional Association for Transgender Health. Available at: https://www.wpath.org/publications/soc. Accessed May 23, 2019.

26. Baker KE, Wilson LM, Sharma R, et al. Hormone therapy, mental health, and quality of life among transgender people: a systematic review. J Endocr Soc 2021;5(4):bvab011.

27. Radix A. Hormone therapy for transgender adults. Urol Clin North Am 2019;46(4):467–73.

28. Coleman E, Radix AE, Bouman WP, et al. Standards of Care for the Health of Transgender and Gender Diverse People, Version 8. Int J Transgender Health 2022;23(sup1):S1–259.

29. Sudhakar D, Huang Z, Zietkowski M, et al. Feminizing gender-affirming hormone therapy for the transgender and gender diverse population: An overview of treatment modality, monitoring, and risks. Neurourol Urodyn 2023;42(5):903–20.
30. Glintborg D, T'Sjoen G, Ravn P, et al. Management of endocrine disease: optimal feminizing hormone treatment in transgender people. Eur J Endocrinol 2021; 185(2):R49–63.
31. Herndon JS, Maheshwari AK, Nippoldt TB, et al. Comparison of the subcutaneous and intramuscular estradiol regimens as part of gender-affirming hormone therapy. Endocr Pract 2023;29(5):356–61.
32. TransLine Hormone Therapy Prescriber Guidelines. TransLine: Transgender Medical Consultation Service. Available at: https://transline.zendesk.com/hc/en-us/articles/229373288-TransLine-Hormone-Therapy-Prescriber-Guidelines. Accessed June 24, 2023.
33. Totaro M, Palazzi S, Castellini C, et al. Risk of venous thromboembolism in transgender people undergoing hormone feminizing therapy: a prevalence meta-analysis and meta-regression study. Front Endocrinol 2021;12:741866.
34. Patibandla S, Heaton J, Kyaw H. Spironolactone. In: StatPearls. StatPearls Publishing; 2023. Available at: http://www.ncbi.nlm.nih.gov/books/NBK554421/. Accessed June 27, 2023.
35. Controlled Substance Schedules. Available at: https://www.deadiversion.usdoj.gov/schedules/. Accessed June 30, 2023.
36. Defreyne J, T'Sjoen G. Transmasculine hormone therapy. Endocrinol Metab Clin North Am 2019;48(2):357–75.
37. Hanley K, Wittenberg H, Gurjala D, et al. Caring for transgender patients: complications of gender-affirming genital surgeries. Ann Emerg Med 2021;78(3): 409–15.
38. Shin SJ, Kumar A, Safer JD. Gender-affirming surgery: perioperative medical care. Endocr Pract 2022;28(4):420–4.
39. Rosendale N, Goldman S, Ortiz GM, et al. Acute clinical care for transgender patients: a review. JAMA Intern Med 2018;178(11):1535–43.
40. Kinney MK, Pearson TE, Ralston Aoki J. Improving "Life Chances": Surveying the Anti-Transgender Backlash, and Offering a Transgender Equity Impact Assessment Tool for Policy Analysis. J Law Med Ethics 2022;50(3):489–508.
41. ANA Rejects Laws and Policies that Allow Health Care Professionals to Discriminate Against LGBTQIA+ Populations. ANA. Published May 23, 2023. Available at: https://www.nursingworld.org/news/news-releases/2023/ana-rejects-laws-against-lgbtq-care/. Accessed March 4, 2024.
42. 2024 Anti-Trans Bills: Trans Legislation Tracker. Available at: https://translegislation.com. Accessed February 26, 2024.
43. Expósito-Campos P, Salaberria K, Pérez-Fernández JI, et al. Gender detransition: A critical review of the literature. Actas Esp Psiquiatr 2023;51(3):98–118.
44. MacKinnon KR, Kia H, Salway T, et al. Health care experiences of patients discontinuing or reversing prior gender-affirming treatments. JAMA Netw Open 2022;5(7):e2224717.

Nurses Supporting Women and Transfeminine Clients Navigating Non-inclusive Standing Orders

Ethan C. Cicero, PhD, RN[a],*, Jess Dillard-Wright, PhD, MA, RN, CNM[b],
Katherine Croft, BSN, RN[c],
Christine Rodriguez, DNP, APRN, FNP-BC, MDiv, MA[d],
Jordon D. Bosse, PhD, RN[e]

KEYWORDS

- Nursing • Gender identity • Transgender • Nonbinary • Gender-affirming
- Inclusive approaches • Clinical judgment

KEY POINTS

- Nurses are under no obligation to implement standing orders without first determining if the order is applicable to the situation and appropriate for the client.
- Non-inclusive standing orders not only can affect how nurses perform assessments and make clinically-informed decisions about their clients and their care, but also can undermine client autonomy, jeopardize their trust and future engagement with the health care system, and adversely impact their health.
- When defining a standing order's client population using sex or gender and either is referenced as a binary distinction, it can result in segments of the population being disregarded or erased. Further, it decreases care efficiency if standing orders do not account for certain demographics, creating a secondary workflow for some client groups that are not represented by the language used within the standing order, which can lead to care being delayed.

Continued

---

[a] Emory University, Nell Hodgson Woodruff School of Nursing, 1520 Clifton Road, Atlanta, GA 30322, USA; [b] Elaine Marieb College of Nursing, University of Massachusetts Amherst, 130 Skinner Hall, 651 North Pleasant Street, Amherst, MA 01103, USA; [c] UNC Health Transgender Health Program, University of North Carolina Medical Center, 101 Manning Drive, Chapel Hill, NC 27514, USA; [d] Yale School of Nursing, Yale University, 400 West Campus Drive, Orange, CT 06477, USA; [e] College of Nursing, University of Rhode Island, 350 Eddy Street, Providence, RI 02903, USA
* Corresponding author.
E-mail address: ethan.cicero@emory.edu

Nurs Clin N Am 59 (2024) 637–654
https://doi.org/10.1016/j.cnur.2024.07.016
0029-6465/24/© 2024 Elsevier Inc. All rights reserved, including those for text and data mining, AI training, and similar technologies.
nursing.theclinics.com

Continued

- Nurses should work with their colleagues in "altering systemic structures that have a negative influence on individual and community health," a key provision in our Code of Ethics. This equates to advocating for care approaches, standing orders, and other institutional policies that are aligned with health care needs and experiences of their clients while containing language that is inclusive to all client populations.

INTRODUCTION

Nurses working in a variety of inpatient and outpatient settings utilize standing orders to guide the assessment, diagnosis, and treatment of specific clinical problems. Standing orders outline parameters of specified situations where a nurse may act and can perform specific duties such as the administration of immunizations, collection of routine laboratories for chronic health condition monitoring, and initiation of diagnostic evaluations or testing. State Boards of Nursing outline statutes and regulations pertaining to standing orders, and in some states standing orders are referred to as "protocols" or "standing protocols,"[1,2] which is an important distinction for nurses to recognize.

The term "order" connotes a hierarchy and an authoritative command that requires subordination. The role of the nurse has evolved from a silent worker tasked with carrying out technical skills to an active member of the care team. As members of the interdisciplinary care team, nurses bring unique knowledge rooted in a combination of clinical, empirical, and conceptual knowledge.[3] Nurses are active participants in the development and implementation of plans of care and apply nursing knowledge throughout the process. With the evolution of the nurse's role, nurses also have an ethical responsibility to question inappropriate or problematic orders.[4] Like any provider order, nurses are under no obligation to implement standing orders without first determining if the order is applicable to the situation and appropriate for the client.

In this article, we present a case study that illustrates the nurse's obligation in applying clinical judgment in determining the appropriateness of carrying out a standing order. The case study also reveals some of the challenges transgender, nonbinary, and other gender expansive (TNGE) people may experience when health care institutions have standing orders that are not inclusive of all gender identities. We describe the experience of a transfeminine person presenting with abdominal pain at an emergency department (ED) and their interactions with a triage nurse. The focus of the case presentation is to highlight how nurses must first use their clinical judgment to determine the applicability and appropriateness of a standing order, and how nurses can navigate institutional policies that reinforce a gender binary and heteronormative ideals of womanhood while depriving the client of their autonomy. As such, the details of the case study and the discussion that follows will concentrate on the clinical encounter and interpersonal interaction between the nurse and client, and not on the clinical characteristics or treatment plan for the client's chief complaint.

Although this case study centers on the experience of a transfeminine person, the scenario we describe is generalizable to other communities such as cisgender girls and women, transmasculine people, and other gender expansive people with childbearing capabilities (those who were assigned female at birth). This case study can be used as an educational tool during monthly nursing unit meetings, grand rounds, and to facilitate a discussion about how to improve the environment and care provided at your institution. We draw upon our collective nursing experience and knowledge about TNGE people interactions with health care in constructing this hypothetical scenario. The case study builds on our article that discussed the essentials for facilitating gender-affirming nursing encounters with TNGE clients,[5] which was published in this journal's special issue, The Culture of Care. As such, we briefly define relevant terms (**Table 1**) before presenting the case study.

Table 1
Terminology associated with transgender, nonbinary, and other gender expansive people

Term	Definition
Cisgender	An adjective that describes people with an alignment between their sex assigned at birth aligns and gender identity.
Gender affirmation	An interpersonal, interactive process where an individual's gender identity or gender expression is socially accepted and supported.
Gender expansive	"An adjective often used to describe people who identify or express themselves in ways that broaden the socially and culturally defined behaviors or beliefs associated with a particular sex."[6(pS252)]
Gender expression	Outward expression of gender through a combination of behaviors and mannerisms that includes name, pronouns, clothing, haircut, voice, body language, and other physical attributes.
Gender identity	A sense of self and their gender: being a man, woman, both, neither, or something else entirely, and it evolves across the lifespan
Nonbinary	An adjective that "refers to those with gender identities outside the gender binary. People with nonbinary gender identities may identify as partially a man and partially a woman or identify as sometimes a man and sometimes a woman, or identify as a gender other than a man or a woman, or as not having a gender at all. Nonbinary people may use the pronouns they/them/theirs instead of he/him/his or she/her/hers. Some nonbinary people consider themselves to be transgender; some do not because they consider transgender to be part of the gender binary. Examples of nonbinary gender identities may include genderqueer, gender diverse, genderfluid, demigender, bigender, and agender." [6(pS252)]
Sex assigned at birth	Sex is determined and assigned at birth based primarily on the appearance of external genitalia. AFAB is an abbreviation for "assigned female at birth." AMAB is an abbreviation for "assigned male at birth."
Transfeminine	An adjective to describe individuals who identify on the feminine gender spectrum and were assigned male at birth.[7]
Transgender	An adjective that describes individuals with a gender identity that does not align with the sex they were assigned at birth.
Transition	"A process whereby people usually change from the gender expression associated with their assigned sex at birth to another gender expression that better matches their gender identity. People may transition socially by using methods such as changing their name, pronoun, clothing, hair styles, and/or the ways that they move and speak. Transitioning may or may not involve hormones and/or surgeries to alter the physical body. Transition can be used to describe the process of changing one's gender expression from any gender to a different gender. People may transition more than once in their lifetimes."[6(pS253)] Transition is not a linear process from one gender to another gender; the only ideal 'endpoint' is what the TNGE person identifies as necessary to feel at home in their body.
Transmasculine	An adjective to describe individuals who identify on the masculine gender spectrum and were assigned female at birth.[7]

Definitions adopted from Cicero EC, Bosse JD, Ducar D, Rodriguez C, Dillard-Wright J. Facilitating gender-affirming nursing encounters. Nurs Clin North Am. 2024;59(1):75-96. https://doi.org/10.1016/j.cnur.2023.11.007.

CASE STUDY

S.P. (she/her) is a 28-year old transfeminine person and graduate student at a local university. S.P. has an established primary care provider who also prescribes and manages her gender-affirming hormone therapy. S.P. began feminizing hormone therapy and underwent breast augmentation surgery approximately 6 years ago.

S.P. presents for care at the ED with a chief complaint of abdominal pain. Upon checking-in at registration, S.P.'s demographic information contained within her electronic health record (EHR), is verified. The sex marker within the EHR as well as on her driver's license and health insurance card all reflect female. A triage nurse welcomes S.P. and brings her into an examination room to obtain a set of vital signs and conduct a brief initial assessment focused on her chief complaint. Through this process, the triage nurse determines that S.P. is stable and classifies her as a least urgent client with a low acuity level. Before continuing with a more detailed assessment and history taking, the triage nurse initiates diagnostic measures as indicated by the hospital's standing order ("*Women that present to the ED with abdominal pain must undergo a human chorionic gonadotropin urine screening test to rule out pregnancy*") to rule out the possibility of pregnancy for this client. The nurse hands the client a urine collection cup and provides her with instructions for the collection of a clean catch urine sample. S.P. asks, "What do you need my urine for?" The nurse responds, "We have to see if you are pregnant. We do this with all women who present to the ED with abdominal pain." S.P. partially smiles and says, "Oh, ok. Right." S.P. wanted to inform the nurse that she was not pregnant, and that it was anatomically impossible, but she was worried about objecting and that her disclosure would affect the care she received in the ED because when she questioned the medical necessity of care approaches during previous health care encounters, she was refused care and experienced negative interactions with health care professionals.

After S.P. returns from the bathroom with her urine sample, the nurse continues the assessment and history taking. During the genitourinary history, the nurse first asks, "When was your last menstrual cycle?" The client hesitates and then explains, "I have not had any." The nurse astonishingly remarks, "Us women, we all at 1 point have menstruated. I understand this may be an uncomfortable topic for many, but I can assure you that any women who enter our ED with abdominal pain are asked this question." The client responds, "I am transgender, and I am not capable of menstruating because I do not have those body parts." The triage nurse, who visibly looks surprised, responds, "Thank you for letting me know. I did not realize you were transgender." The nurse then advises the client that the triage process is complete, and she will soon be further assessed by a primary nurse once a treatment room is available. S.P. is brought back to the waiting area and the nurse sends the collected urine specimen to the laboratory for analysis without considering the information S.P. provided during the encounter. The nurse did not conduct a sexual health history or ask the client if they could be pregnant.

DISCUSSION OF CASE STUDY

This case study describes the experiences of a transfeminine person presenting with abdominal pain at an ED, one of the most common reasons why adults seek care at an ED.[8] It also exposes a critical failure of the triage nurse to properly evaluate the necessity of implementing the standing order as well as systemic and structural issues that nurses and TNGE clients experience when health care institutions have standing orders that are not inclusive of all gender identities. Non-inclusive standing orders can not only affect how nurses perform assessments and make clinically informed decisions about their clients and their care, but can also undermine client autonomy and jeopardizes their trust and future engagement with the health care system.[9] In the discussion that follows, we highlight the relevance of ED care for TNGE clients, examine nursing's ethical obligations relative to the care of all clients, and critically examine the triage nurse's missteps in applying clinical judgment. We address the learning opportunities presented within the case study by offering approaches that nurses can incorporate into their practice. Additionally, we scrutinize the exclusionary language and faulty assumptions that shape the standing order presented in the case study. And finally, we describe actions nurses should take within their institutions when facing similar challenges related to problematic standing orders.

Relevance of Inclusive Emergency Department Care for Transgender, Nonbinary, and Other Gender Expansive Clients

Nurses interact with and care for TNGE clients in every health care environment. Sometimes this care entails primary and preventative health care such as immunizations, diagnostic testing, or the initiation and/or continuation of gender-affirming hormone therapy. Other times, care might include a visit to the ED for more acute and emergent health concerns. It is worth noting that multi-level barriers to accessing affirming health care may mean the ED sometimes serves as a primary health care site for some TNGE people,[10] and TNGE people are more likely to seek health care in an ED than cisgender people.[11] Regardless of cause, TNGE people access the ED for a variety of health concerns that are unrelated to their TNGE status, but their identities should be accounted for in how nursing care is delivered.

Nurses Ethical Commitments

As nurses, our commitment to our clients and their health is outlined in the American Nurses Association Code of Ethics[4]; nursing care must be delivered with "compassion and respect for the inherent dignity, worth, and unique attributes of every person."[4(p1)] Furthermore, nurses are responsible to assure that the appropriate care is provided to optimize the health and well-being of their clients, which includes "acting to minimize unwarranted, unwanted, or unnecessary medical treatment."[4(p2)] The nurse in the case study treated the client with respect, but they did not recognize the importance of documenting the client's gender identity within the EHR. With this documentation, other health care professionals caring for this client at this hospital will be better equipped in providing person-centered and appropriate care. The nurse in the case study should have navigated this responsibility in partnership with the client. After the client disclosed their transgender status, an affirming response by the nurse would be:

> I can update your chart, so it reflects your current gender identity. Here are all the options we have in our system, which one best describes your current gender: man, woman, transgender woman, transgender man, nonbinary, or something else? And for something else, I can type in the term you use to describe yourself.

Health care providers may be hesitant to collect sexual orientation and gender identity (SOGI) data in the ED, but research suggests that the majority of clients are willing to share this information.[12]

Nurses and other health care professionals must consider how the client's gender identity affects their care and treatment plan. Nurses may need to ask additional and relevant health history questions and apply clinical judgment when considering which assessments and diagnostic procedures are necessary and appropriate for their client. It is quite possible that the triage nurse was unfamiliar with TNGE health topics beyond the training they received at their hospital on collecting SOGI data, despite not asking about or documenting the client's sexual orientation. Nurses should seek out additional education pertaining to the client populations they serve. Understanding core concepts of gender-affirming care and related medical interventions as well as the health consequences stemming from receiving non-affirming health care, experiencing discrimination, and enduring the politicization of TNGE bodies and their human rights will create a stronger, more capable and effective nurse and client advocate.[5] See **Table 2** for educational resources on TNGE health topics.

Table 2
TNGE health and educational resources
Nurses are receiving more education, either at the prelicensure level or as professionals via continuing education, on caring for TNGE clients.[1] However, many of these efforts are taking place in individual programs and institutions rather than being implemented into nursing curricula broadly. It is often delivered within a single course or as a standalone presentation that concentrates on gender-affirming medical interventions such as hormone therapy and surgical procedures.[13] These presentations are frequently peppered with deficit-framed statistics about the health inequities experienced by the TNGE population, fixated on suicidality, substance use, and sexually transmitted infections. While these are real and important TNGE health topics, they do not encompass the depth and breadth of TNGE care and thus should not exemplify the depth and breadth of nursing education provided on TNGE health. This kind of cursory treatment of TNGE health does not prepare nurses to provide appropriate, equitable, and affirming care to TNGE people. It also centers nurses as not TNGE people and "others" TNGE folks. Below are resources nurses can use to supplement their knowledge base about TNGE individuals and their health.

Organization	Description
GLMA: Health Professionals Advancing LGBTQ + Equality	Professional association of LGBTQ+ and allied health professionals, which includes a Nursing Section. They focus on research, advocacy, and education. GLMA offers webinars, conferences, online educational modules, an LGBTQ + friendly provider list, and resources for LGBTQ + clients. www.glma.org
Human Rights Campaign Health Care Equality Index	Guidance on policies and practices that is inclusive of LGBTQ + clients, visitors, and employees, with specific resources available for Veteran's and Children's hospitals. https://www.thehrcfoundation.org/professional-resources/hei-resource-guide Institutions can also apply for recognition for their inclusive policies through the Health Care Equality Index https://www.thehrcfoundation.org/professional-resources/hei-scoring-criteria
Lambda Legal	Creating Equal Access to Quality Health Care for Transgender Patients: Transgender-Affirming Hospital Policies https://legacy.lambdalegal.org/publications/fs_transgender-affirming-hospital-policies
National LGBT Health Education Center at The Fenway Institute	National LGBT Health Education Center, hosts annual "Advancing Excellence in Transgender Health" Conference; resources for clients and providers https://fenwayhealth.org/the-fenway-institute/education/the-national-lgbtia-health-education-center/

(continued on next page)

Table 2 (continued)	
Organization	**Description**
Sexual Orientation and Gender Identity Nursing	Created by an interdisciplinary group of professionals and academics from Canada, the website is a toolkit for nurses and nursing educators committed to providing resources and education in health care. https://soginursing.ca
Transgender Training Institute	Guide to pronouns. https://www.transgendertraininginstitute.com/resources/pronouns/
UCSF Gender Affirming Health Program	Publishes the "Guidelines for the primary and gender-affirming care of transgender and gender nonbinary people" https://transcare.ucsf.edu/guidelines and hosts the biannual conference, "National Transgender Health Summit" https://prevention.ucsf.edu/transhealth
World Professional Association for Transgender Health	An international, multidisciplinary, professional association that promotes evidence-based care, education, research, public policy, and respect in transgender health. www.wpath.org

Adopted from Cicero EC, Bosse JD, Ducar D, Rodriguez C, Dillard-Wright J. Facilitating gender-affirming nursing encounters. Nurs Clin North Am. 2024;59(1):75-96. https://doi.org/10.1016/j.cnur.2023.11.007.

Clinical Judgment and Point-of-Care Improvements

Clinical judgment, one of the key attributes of professional nursing, requires critical thinking, clinical reasoning, and nursing knowledge.[14] The nurse in the case study failed to apply clinical judgment in determining the appropriateness of carrying out the standing order. The nurse only determined that the order was applicable to the situation—S.P. is a woman who presented to the ED with abdominal pain. However, by failing to conduct a sexual health history, asking the client directly if they could be pregnant, or applying the knowledge gained from the client disclosing their TNGE status and the absence of reproductive organs required for pregnancy, the nurse neglected to determine if the order was appropriate for the client.

Clinical decisions are grounded by clinical judgment and are associated with care outcomes.[14] For S.P., an unnecessary pregnancy screen may seem innocuous, and aside from the additional and unwarranted health care expense, the interaction with the nurse and specimen collection may have a detrimental impact on the client's mental health. Discussions of infertility with all patients should be handled with care and sensitivity. An individual who desires pregnancy and is unable to achieve it may experience negative feelings and other psychological sequelae in response to this experience. In this case study, achieving pregnancy is anatomically impossible for S.P., a conclusion the triage nurse should have been able to draw from the client's gender identity. For some clients, like S.P., obtaining a clinical history may be sufficient to rule out pregnancy; other clinical circumstances include history of hysterectomy or tubal ligation. Other client populations that may experience negative health outcomes from encountering a similar scenario include.

- Client populations with pregnancy desires, regardless of gender, such as cisgender women with infertility challenges or those who require intrauterine or artificial insemination or assisted reproductive technology (ART) procedures such as in vitro fertilization or embryo transfers as well transgender women or transfeminine persons who experience gender dysphoria and distress related to infertility or lack of childbearing capability.

- Cisgender women who engage in sex with other individuals that have childbearing potential (eg, cisgender women, transgender men, transmasculine people, nonbinary folks assigned female at birth) will not become pregnant without techniques such as intrauterine insemination or ART procedures. Assuming that every woman or female-presenting client is cisgender and engages in intercourse that could result in pregnancy and without assessing the client's sexual health history can lead to inappropriate care. Further, failing to apply the knowledge gained from a comprehensive assessment can also be emotionally distressing to clients.
- Some transgender men, transmasculine people, nonbinary people, and other gender expansive folks can become pregnant. Failing to perform necessary diagnostic testing may be detrimental to their client's life.[15] Worth noting, gender-affirming hormone therapy is not a substitute for contraception[7]; TNGE people taking masculinizing hormones can still get pregnant and TNGE individuals taking feminizing hormones continue to produce viable sperm.[7]

Standing orders, like the one featured in the case study, are often in place and performed prior to anesthesia, surgery, and diagnostic radiography due to the potential risk for fetal harm.[16,17] While the American Society of Anesthesiologists (ASA) recommends pregnancy screening, they explain it should not be considered a mandatory test[16]; informed consent should be obtained to respect the client's autonomy.[16] The American College of Radiology (ACR) outlines 2 components that can determine pregnancy status: clinical history and pregnancy testing.[17]

Organ Inventories and Inclusive Sexual Health Histories

Appropriate health and sexual health questions can help eliminate unnecessary pregnancy screenings. In addition to SOGI collection, by maintaining an organ inventory (**Box 1**) for all clients, nurses and other health care professionals are better equipped in their decision-making and the delivery of appropriate person-centered care.

Box 1
Organ inventory

What is it?
An organ inventory involves charting the presence or absence of specific organs; data should be collected from all clients and updated at least annually.[18,19]

Why should we collect it?
Nurses can use the information to make informed decisions about the relevance and necessity of diagnostic tests and provide clients with recommendations for needed preventative screenings.

For example, if an individual has breasts and a cervix, regardless of how they identify, they should undergo an age-appropriate breast cancer screening with mammograms and cervical cancer screenings with a Papanicolaou test (Pap). However, an individual with breasts but no cervix will only require age-appropriate breast cancer screenings with mammograms.[6]

Obtaining a sexual health history is critical when individuals with child-bearing potential presents with abdominal pain. All clients have diverse sexual identities, sexual partnerships, and practices, and sometimes, the client's sexual orientation may not align with their sexual behaviors.[15] An inclusive and affirming approach that is grounded in trauma-informed care is necessary and will help facilitate the collection of clinically relevant and accurate information from the client, and inform diagnostic and treatment plans. **Table 3** provides an approach to conducting an inclusive sexual health history, which was adopted from the Centers for Disease Control and Prevention (CDC)[20] and the National LGBTQIA + Health Education Center.[21] It represents key areas nurses should discuss with their clients, and nurses may need to ask follow-up questions and additional questions relevant to the clinical circumstances.

Table 3
Conducting an inclusive sexual health history

Aspect of the Assessment	Example Questions	Nursing Implications
Prior to the assessment, garner consent from the client.	• May I ask you a few questions about your sexual health and sexual practices? I understand that these questions are personal, but they are important for your overall health. • I ask these questions to all my patients, regardless of age, gender, or marital status. These questions are as important as the questions about other areas of your physical and mental health. This information is kept in strict confidence unless you or someone else is being hurt or is in danger. Do you have any questions before we get started?	• Some clients may be uncomfortable when discussing their sexual health history. They may have experienced sexual abuse, violence, or trauma in their lives or within a health care environment. To help establish a therapeutic nursing relationship with all clients, nurses should use a trauma-informed approach when conducting any assessment, particularly a sexual health history.[5] • When possible, conduct as much of the sexual health history while the client is clothed.[15] • Never make assumptions about the client's sexual orientation, gender identity, or the gender identity of their sexual partner(s).
Preferences	• What language do you use to refer to your body (ie, genitals)? • Are you currently sexually active?	• Mirror the language used by the client whenever possible, and ask for clarification if the client uses unfamiliar language. • When the client's chosen language can't be used for any reason, using broad language like "groin" with descriptors like "internal" and "external" can be helpful.[12]
Partners	• Are you sexually active with one partner or more than one? • How would your partners identify themselves in terms of gender?	• Refrain from asking clients, "Are you sexually active with men, women, or both?" This approach inaccurately assumes that gender is binary.

(continued on next page)

Table 3 (continued)		
Aspect of the Assessment	**Example Questions**	**Nursing Implications**
	• Do you or your partner(s) currently have other sex partners? • Is it possible that any of your sex partners in the past year had sex with someone else while they were still in a sexual relationship with you?	Instead, ask clients about the gender(s) of their partner(s). • If the client uses the terms "man" or "woman" when describing the gender of their partner(s), the nurse should verify if the client is referring to cisgender, transgender, or nonbinary identified partners. • Never assume that a client's previously documented sexual orientation or a client's partner status is still accurate. Similarly, nurses should not be alarmed if a client's recent sexual behavior does not align with their (previously) stated sexual orientation. • If a client has had sex in the past, but is not currently, it is still important to take a sexual history.
Practices	• What kind of sexual contact do you have, or have you had? What parts of your body are involved when you have sex? (eg, oral sex, vaginal sex, anal sex, sharing sex toys) • Do you use toys inside your [insert preferred language for genitals] or anus, or do you use them on your partners? • Do you have any other types of sex that hasn't been asked about?	• Asking about sex practices will guide the assessment of client risk, risk-reduction strategies, and the determination of necessary testing. • Focus on the information you need to know based on what you have already learned about the patient. • Do not assume that all primary and secondary sexual characteristics correspond to the stated gender(s) of their partner(s). Instead, ask about what specific anatomy for the client and their partner(s) are used during sexual encounters.[15]

(continued on next page)

Table 3 (continued)		
Aspect of the Assessment	Example Questions	Nursing Implications
Protection from STIs	• What do you do to protect yourself from HIV and STIs? • Tell me about when you use condoms or other prevention tools. • There are a lot of reasons why people don't use condoms or other barriers or prevention tools. Can you tell me why you are not using them for sex? • When was the last time you had unprotected sex?	• Nurses should determine the appropriate level of risk-reduction education for each client. • Provide education on testing and prevention methods to clients at risk for STIs, including information about pre-exposure prophylaxis (PrEP) for individuals at high risk for contracting HIV.
Past history of STIs	• Have you been diagnosed with an STI in the past? When? Did you get treatment? Have you had any symptoms that keep coming back? • Has your current partner or any former partners ever been diagnosed or treated for an STI? Were you tested for the same STI(s)? Do you know your partner(s) HIV status?	• A history of prior STIs may place the client at greater risk now. • Provide STI prevention and treatment education to client.
Pregnancy intention	• When you are having sex, is there any exposure to sperm or chance of pregnancy? • Do you have any plans or desires to have (more) children?	• In addition to sexual behavior, pregnancy intention and desire are important considerations to keep in mind if the client requires a pregnancy screen.
Partner violence	• Has anyone ever forced or compelled you to do anything sexually that you did not want to do? • Is there any violence in any of your relationships? • Have you experienced physical, sexual, or emotional violence from a partner?	If a client discloses a traumatic event: 1. Listen 2. Communicate belief, "That must have been frightening to you." 3. Emphasize the unacceptability of violence, "Violence is unacceptable. I'm sorry that happened, that should not have happened." 4. Be clear that the client is not to blame, "What happened is not your fault." 5. Make a safety plan/provide resources

Adopted from the CDC[20] and the National LGBTQIA + Health Education Center.[21] The information provided in the table represents areas nurses should discuss with their clients, and nurses may need to ask follow-up questions and additional questions relevant to the clinical circumstances.

Additional Point-of-Care Improvements

Often within an ED, nurses collect biological samples from their clients before completing a focused assessment and determining which diagnostic tests are needed. In the case study, the nurse treated the urine collection as part of a cascade of tasks that needed to be performed as part of the patient assessment, overlooking the client's autonomy. It is critical for nurses to discuss the purpose for the collection and what types of tests or screenings will be conducted on their sample(s). The nurse can also remind the individual that they have control over what happens to their body and that they have the right to refuse any test or screening. At the same time, the nurse should clearly explain whether refusing a particular test or screening will have an impact on care decisions or the subsequent care delivered (eg, if requiring a pregnancy test as a criteria for having surgery, not doing so could jeopardize their ability to have the surgery).

We recognize that nurses cannot change institutional standing orders while actively caring for clients, and that even when changes are in progress, they can take time. In the case study, if the client asserted that the pregnancy screening was not necessary or if they refused the test, the nurse should reassess if in fact the standing order is applicable to the situation and appropriate for the client. If the nurse considered the client's feedback and concerns, asked additional and relevant health history questions, they may have determined that the order was not appropriate for the client. Once the nurse correctly determined that the standing order was not appropriate to carry out, they should document the reasons substantiating their decision within the EHR and pass on their decision as part of their report to the next person who will be providing care. Actions that can be taken to address the issue more systematically will be discussed further.

Exclusionary Language and Faulty Assumptions of Standing Orders

Standing orders can improve efficiency and expedite health care decision making. Important components of effective standing orders include clear delineation for who is responsible for each task and describing the patient or client population to whom the order applies.[22] Client populations are often defined using diagnostic criteria such as "persons diagnosed with diabetes," by discrete patient complaints or conditions such as "individuals presenting with chest pain," and can further be specified using demographic characteristics as in "women with abdominal pain." When defining a client population using sex or gender and either is referenced as a binary distinction, it can result in segments of the population, being disregarded or erased.[15,23-25] Further, it decreases care efficiency if standing orders do not account for certain demographics, creating a secondary workflow for some client groups that are not represented by the language used within the standing order, which can lead to care being delayed.

The standing order presented in the case study contains exclusionary language and is grounded with faulty assumptions that are in direct opposition to both clinical reality and scientific evidence. For example, using the term "women" is not an inclusive approach to define a client population because it is not inclusive of all applicable gender identities and is subjective of what constitutes the intended client population. This approach results in segments of the population being disregarded or erased, particularly transgender women and transfeminine people.[15,23-25] Standing orders should clearly define the client population and relative clinical conditions. Using language such as "individuals of child-bearing potential" or "women and others with child-bearing potential" reflects more inclusive and accurate terminology. Below, in **Table 4**, we highlight some key examples of the assumptions contained within the standing order.

Table 4
Faulty assumptions in the case study's standing order

Assumption	Reality
Only and all women can become pregnant.	Some transgender men, nonbinary people, and other gender expansive folks can become pregnant, and some cisgender women do not have child-bearing potential due to infertility, sexual behaviors and practices, surgical history, and/or present anatomy. Worth noting, gender-affirming hormone therapy is not a substitute for contraception[6]; TNGE people taking masculinizing hormones can still get pregnant and TNGE individuals taking feminizing hormones continue to produce viable sperm.[6] Further reliance on standing order algorithmic logic incentives nurses to lean toward missing populations who could be affected by pregnancy who do not identify as women. This is a situation with arguably a greater chance of harm based on missed diagnostic information that could lead to faster, more efficient, and appropriate treatment.[15]
Child-bearing potential is not considered or deemed necessary for assessment.	Achieving pregnancy can be a complicated process, however, an individual's age, current anatomy, and activities that result in the joining of a sperm with an egg are more valid indicators of child-bearing potential than an individual's gender or gender identity, which can evolve across the lifespan.
People with child-bearing potential possess a uniform desire to become pregnant.	Not all women or TNGE people with child-bearing potential have pregnancy desires, and assuming so can have a detrimental impact on a client's mental health. An individual who desires pregnancy and is unable to achieve it may experience negative feelings in response to this unnecessary test.
Requiring every person with child-bearing potential tested for pregnancy denotes a generalization to the heteronormative and patriarchal notion that a "man" is responsible for impregnating a "woman."	Cisgender women who engage in sex with other individuals that have child-bearing potential (eg, cisgender women, transgender men, transmasculine people, nonbinary folks assigned female at birth) will not become pregnant without intrauterine or artificial insemination or ART procedures such as in vitro fertilization or embryo transfers.
Women are unreliable in predicting their pregnancy status	Obtaining a sexual history and directly asking the client about their pregnancy status are approaches that are highly effective as pregnancy predictors.[17,26] In a study conducted by Strote and Chen examining clients' reliability to predict their pregnancy status,[26] 130 clients stated that they were not sexually active and were not pregnant; urine and serum pregnancy tests confirmed this self-report and determined all were not pregnant. Among 336 patients that stated that there was no chance they could be pregnant, there was a 99.7% negative predictive value.[26] However, researchers suggest pregnancy screening is appropriate for clients who are unsure of their pregnancy status, a practice that is recommended by the ASA as well as the ACR and Centers for Disease Control and Prevention.[16,17,27]

Nurses Addressing the Institution—From Individual to Collective Action

Nurses should work with their colleagues in "altering systemic structures that have a negative influence on individual and community health,"[4(p2)] a key provision in our Code of Ethics. This equates to advocating for care approaches, standing orders, and other institutional policies that are aligned with health care needs and experiences of their clients while containing language that is inclusive to all client populations. Nurses have an ethical responsibility to advocate for change at the institutional level once they recognize a standing order contains problematic language or is grounded with faulty assumptions. Nursing shared governance is a helpful structure through which to take action.

Nursing shared governance

Shared governance is a model that includes the input of nurses providing direct care at all levels of the organization, ranging from unit-specific projects to identify and implement process improvements in care delivery to the formulation of organization-wide goals.[28] Ideally, shared governance empowers nurses on the front lines with the autonomy and authority to *act* in ways that support clinical excellence.[29] Successful shared governance also includes promoting multidisciplinary involvement.[30]

Let us imagine the nurse in the case study presents their concern about the standing order to the ED's shared governance committee. Then, if the committee agrees with the nurse's concern, a systematic plan would be used to implement and evaluate any proposed changes. One commonly used framework that involves an iterative process is the "Plan, Do, Study, Act" (PDSA) cycle.[31] Below, we provide an example of how the PDSA cycle could be applied to make iterative changes to the standing order and evaluate the process (**Table 5**).

Table 5
Applying the PDSA cycle to advocate for systemic change

PDSA Cycle	Example of Action
Plan. Obtain input from stakeholders, including the nurses who will be implementing the changes.	• Obtained input from staff nurses and members of the TNGE community to identify specific language in the standing order that can be changed for a more inclusive and appropriately worded standing order. • Advocated to change "women that present to the ED" to "individuals with child-bearing potential that present to the ED." This revision reflects inclusive and accurate language. • Reviewing best practices for working with TNGE populations,[6] the group decided that specific assessment approaches and questions (eg, sexual health history, organ inventory; see **Box 1, Table 3**) will be referenced in the new standing order. This addition will ensure that nurses are better equipped in their decision-making and the delivery of appropriate person-centered care. • Trained ED nurses about the new standing order and assessment questions, with the rationale for the changes.

(continued on next page)

Table 5 (*continued*)	
PDSA Cycle	**Example of Action**
Do. Implement the change(s) in a single unit for a short period of time.	The new standing order and any relevant nursing assessments were described to the ED nurses. For the next 3 months, the ED nurses worked with the new assessment and standing orders, and noted any challenges in the monthly unit shared governance meetings.
Study. Re-group in 3 months to evaluate the change: What was learned, what went well, what improvements can be made?	At the end of 3 months, the group met and gathered the notes from the monthly shared governance meetings and additional feedback from the front line nurses and the prescribing providers were collated and reviewed.
Act. Use data to determine whether to permanently implement the change(s) or whether additional revisions are necessary.	• The shared governance committee brought in information technology professionals with the capability of creating new fields in the EHR to allow for clear documentation of assigned sex at birth, gender, pronouns, as well inclusive sexual and reproductive health history-taking. • Nurses appreciated the inclusion of specific assessment approaches and clinical questions to the standing order. The addition of an organ inventory allowed the nursing staff to quickly identify which clients were not capable of achieving pregnancy. Nurses reported feeling empowered, able to function to their fullest capacity, and apply clinical judgment and to determine whether a pregnancy screening was necessary. The referenced items will appear as links that takes the EHR user to the referenced item's field/form within the EHR system. • Once the nurses and other stakeholders were satisfied with the processes, a final version of the order was drafted. As part of the final revision process, the committee reviewed State Board of Nursing guidelines for what needs to be included in a standing order and how frequently it must be reviewed, as these requirements may vary from state to state.

SUMMARY

In addition to outlining parameters of specified situations where a nurse can act and perform specific duties without having to first obtain a provider order, standing orders should also be person-centered, reflect the current body of knowledge, and empower nurses to make clinically-sound decisions rooted in appropriate assessments and in the delivery of trauma-informed care. The use of exclusionary language in standing orders related to gender can contribute to ineffective use of clinical judgment, unnecessary health care expenses, and screenings, and in some cases, can result in misdiagnosis or direct patient harm, either physically or emotionally. Nurses are responsible in assuring that the appropriate care is provided to optimize the health and well-being of their clients, which includes "acting to minimize unwarranted, unwanted, or unnecessary medical treatment" and "altering systemic structures that have a negative influence on individual and community health."[4(p2)] Nurses who work in institutions with standing orders in place that do not reflect the needs of the clients can advocate for change as part of nurses' commitment to deliver care with "compassion and respect for the inherent dignity, worth, and unique attributes of every person."[4(p1)]

CLINICS CARE POINTS

- Nurses need to be familiar with core concepts of gender affirming care, related medical interventions, and health consequences of discrimination, receipt of non-affirming care, and the politicization of TNGE bodies. Nurses who have not received this training in school or through other professional development opportunities should seek out additional education in these areas.

- Nurses and other health care professionals must consider how the client's gender identity affects their care and treatment plan. Nurses may need to ask additional and relevant health history questions and apply clinical judgment when considering which assessments and diagnostic procedures are necessary and appropriate for their client.

- Nurses should work with their colleagues in "altering systemic structures that have a negative influence on individual and community health," a key provision in our Code of Ethics. This equates to advocating for care approaches, standing orders, and other institutional policies that are aligned with health care needs and experiences of their clients while containing language that is inclusive to all client populations.

DISCLOSURE

Dr E.C. Cicero was supported by grants from the Alzheimer's Association (23AARGD-NTF-1028973), The National Institute on Alcohol Abuse and Alcoholism (R01AA030275), and the National Institute on Aging (K23AG084851). Dr J.D. Bosse was partially supported by a career development grant funded by the National Center for Complementary and Integrative Health (K01AT012495). The statements in this article are solely the responsibility of the author and do not necessarily represent the views of the Alzheimer's Association or the National Institutes of Health.

REFERENCES

1. North Carolina Board of Nursing. Standing Orders. Position Statement for RN and LPN Practice. 2022. Available at: https://www.ncbon.com/myfiles/downloads/boarsinformation/laws-rules/position-statements/ps-standing-orders.pdf.
2. Massachusetts Board of Registration in Nursing. Accepting, Verifying, Transcribing and Implementing Prescriber Orders 2014. Available at: https://www.google.com/url?sa=t&source=web&rct=j&opi=89978449&url=https://www.mass.gov/files/documents/2018/01/02/AR%25209324%2520Accepting%252C%2520Verifying%252C%2520transcribing%2520and%2520Implementing%2520Prescriber%2520Orders%2520revised%252010-9-14.docx%23:~:text%3DStanding%2520orders%252Fprotocols%2520include%2520written,be%2520implemented%2520by%2520the%2520nurse.&ved=2ahUKEwjZ4q6H3qOFAxVCGVkFHZKDBB0QFnoECA4QAw&usg=AOvVaw0FGpKpWXuAeoBFE989kC6k. Accessed March 31, 2024.
3. Schultz PR, Meleis AI. Nursing epistemology: Traditions, insights, questions. J Nurs Scholarsh 1988;20(4):217–21.

4. American Nurses Association. Code of Ethics for Nurses with Interpretive Statements. 2nd edition. American Nurses Association 2015;64. Available at: https://www.nursingworld.org/practice-policy/nursing-excellence/ethics/code-of-ethics-for-nurses/. Accessed March 1, 2024.

5. Cicero EC, Bosse JD, Ducar D, et al. Facilitating gender-affirming nursing encounters. Nurs Clin North Am. 2024;59(1):75–96. https://doi.org/10.1016/j.cnur.2023.11.007.

6. Coleman E, Radix AE, Bouman WP, et al. Standards of care for the health of transgender and gender diverse people, version 8. Int J Transgend Health 2022; 23(sup 1):S1–259. https://doi.org/10.1080/26895269.2022.2100644.

7. Reisner SL, Radix A, Deutsch MB. Integrated and gender-affirming transgender clinical care and research. J Acquir Immune Defic Syndr 2016;72:S235–42. https://doi.org/10.1097/qai.0000000000001088.

8. Cairns C, Kang K. National hospital ambulatory medical care survey: 2021 emergency department summary tables. 2021. Available at: https://www.cdc.gov/nchs/data/nhamcs/web_tables/2021-nhamcs-ed-web-tables-508.pdf.

9. Cicero EC, Reisner SL, Silva SG, et al. Health care experiences of transgender adults: An integrated mixed research literature review. ANS Adv Nurs Sci. 2019;42(2):123–38.

10. Cruz TM. Assessing access to care for transgender and gender nonconforming people: A consideration of diversity in combating discrimination. Soc Sci Med 2014;110:65–73.

11. Babbs G, Hughto JMW, Shireman TI, et al. Emergency department use disparities among transgender and cisgender medicare beneficiaries, 2011-2020. JAMA Intern Med 2024;184(4):443–5.

12. Bosse JD, Nesteby JA, Randall CE. Integrating sexual minority health issues into a health assessment class. J Prof Nurs 2015;31(6):498–507.

13. Lim F, Ozkara San E. Methods of teaching transgender health in undergraduate nursing programs: A narrative review. Nurse Educ 2023. https://doi.org/10.1097/NNE.0000000000001558.

14. American Association of Colleges of Nursing. Clinical Judgement. Available at: https://www.aacnnursing.org/essentials/tool-kit/domains-concepts/clinical-judgement. Accessed March 25, 2024.

15. Moseson H, Zazanis N, Goldberg E, et al. The imperative for transgender and gender nonbinary inclusion: Beyond women's health. Obstet Gynecol 2020; 135(5):1059–68.

16. American Society of Anesthesiologists, Committee on Quality Management and Departmental Administration. Statement on Pregnancy Testing Prior to Anesthesia and Surgery. Available at: https://www.asahq.org/standards-and-practice-parameters/statement-on-pregnancy-testing-prior-to-anesthesia-and-surgery. Accessed February 12, 2024.

17. American College of Radiology. ACR-SPR Practice Parameter for Imaging Pregnant or Potentially Pregnant Patients with Ionizing Radiation (Resolution 31). Available at: https://www.acr.org/-/media/acr/files/practice-parameters/pregnant-pts.pdf. Accessed February 15, 2024.

18. Kronk CA, Everhart AR, Ashley F, et al. Transgender data collection in the electronic health record: Current concepts and issues. J Am Med Inf Assoc 2022; 29(2):271–84.

19. Grasso C, Goldhammer H, Thompson J, et al. Optimizing gender-affirming medical care through anatomical inventories, clinical decision support, and

population health management in electronic health record systems. J Am Med Inf Assoc 2021;28(11):2531–5.

20. Reno H, Park I, Workowski K, et al. A Guide to Taking a Sexual History. Centers for Disease Control and Prevention; 2022. Available at: https://www.cdc.gov/std/treatment/sexualhistory.htm. Accessed March 25, 2024.

21. Thompson J. Taking a Sexual History with Sexual and Gender Minority Individuals. National LGBTQIA+ Health Education Center; 2020. Available at: https://fenwayhealth.org/wp-content/uploads/6.-Taking-an-Affirming-Sexual-History.pdf. Accessed March 25, 2024.

22. Leubner J, Wild S. Developing standing orders to help your team work to the highest level. Fam Pract Manag 2018;25(3):13–6.

23. Namaste V. Invisible lives: the erasure of transsexual and transgendered people. University of Chicago Press; 2000.

24. Crawford J, Schultz A, Chernomas WM. Interpersonal transphobia within nursing: A critical concept exploration. ANS Adv Nurs Sci. 2023;1–17. https://doi.org/10.1097/ANS.0000000000000491.

25. Bauer GR, Hammond R, Travers R, et al. "I don't think this is theoretical; this is our lives": How erasure impacts health care for transgender people. J Assoc Nurses AIDS Care 2009;20(5):348–61.

26. Strote J, Chen G. Patient self assessment of pregnancy status in the emergency department. Emerg Med J 2006;23(7):554–7.

27. Division of Reproductive Health, National Center for Chronic Disease Prevention and Health Promotion. How to be reasonably certain that a woman is not pregnant. Available at: https://www.cdc.gov/reproductivehealth/contraception/mmwr/spr/notpregnant.html. Accessed March 1, 2024.

28. Hess RG Jr. Professional governance: Another new concept? J Nurs Adm 2017;47(1):1–2.

29. Winslow S, Hougan A, DeGuzman P, et al. The voice of the nurse... What's being said about shared governance? Nurs Manag 2015;46(4):46–51.

30. Nantz S. How to increase unit-based shared governance participation and empowerment. Am Nurse Today 2015;10(1):52–4.

31. Moen RD, Norman C. Clearing up myths about the Deming cycle and seeing how it keeps evolving. Qual Prog 2010;43:22–8.

1. Publication Title	2. Publication Number	3. Filing Date
NURSING CLINICS OF NORTH AMERICA	598 – 960	9/18/2024

4. Issue Frequency	5. Number of Issues Published Annually	6. Annual Subscription Price
MAR, JUN, SEP, DEC	4	$168.00

7. Complete Mailing Address of Known Office of Publication (Not printer) (Street, city, county, state, and ZIP+4®)

ELSEVIER INC.
230 Park Avenue, Suite 800
New York, NY 10169

Contact Person: Malathi Samayan
Telephone (Include area code): 91-44-4299-4507

8. Complete Mailing Address of Headquarters or General Business Office of Publisher (Not printer)

ELSEVIER INC.
230 Park Avenue, Suite 800
New York, NY 10169

9. Full Names and Complete Mailing Addresses of Publisher, Editor, and Managing Editor (Do not leave blank)

Publisher (Name and complete mailing address)

DOLORES MELONI, ELSEVIER INC.
1600 JOHN F KENNEDY BLVD. SUITE 1600
PHILADELPHIA, PA 19103-2899

Editor (Name and complete mailing address)

KERRY HOLLAND, ELSEVIER INC.
1600 JOHN F KENNEDY BLVD. SUITE 1600
PHILADELPHIA, PA 19103-2899

Managing Editor (Name and complete mailing address)

PATRICK MANLEY, ELSEVIER INC.
1600 JOHN F KENNEDY BLVD. SUITE 1600
PHILADELPHIA, PA 19103-2899

10. Owner (Do not leave blank. If the publication is owned by a corporation, give the name and address of the corporation immediately followed by the names and addresses of all stockholders owning or holding 1 percent or more of the total amount of stock. If not owned by a corporation, give the names and addresses of the individual owners. If owned by a partnership or other unincorporated firm, give its name and address as well as those of each individual owner. If the publication is published by a nonprofit organization, give its name and address.)

Full Name	Complete Mailing Address
WHOLLY OWNED SUBSIDIARY OF REED/ELSEVIER, US HOLDINGS	1600 JOHN F KENNEDY BLVD. SUITE 1600 PHILADELPHIA, PA 19103-2899

11. Known Bondholders, Mortgagees, and Other Security Holders Owning or Holding 1 Percent or More of Total Amount of Bonds, Mortgages, or Other Securities. If none, check box ▶ ☐ None

Full Name	Complete Mailing Address
N/A	

12. Tax Status (For completion by nonprofit organizations authorized to mail at nonprofit rates) (Check one)
The purpose, function, and nonprofit status of this organization and the exempt status for federal income tax purposes.
☒ Has Not Changed During Preceding 12 Months
☐ Has Changed During Preceding 12 Months (Publisher must submit explanation of change with this statement)

PS Form **3526**, July 2014 (Page 1 of 4 (see instructions page 4)) PSN 7530-01-000-9931   PRIVACY NOTICE: See our privacy policy on www.usps.com.

---

13. Publication Title	14. Issue Date for Circulation Data Below
NURSING CLINICS OF NORTH AMERICA	JUNE 2024

15. Extent and Nature of Circulation		Average No. Copies Each Issue During Preceding 12 Months	No. Copies of Single Issue Published Nearest to Filing Date
a. Total Number of Copies (Net press run)		189	170
b. Paid Circulation (By Mail and Outside the Mail)	(1) Mailed Outside-County Paid Subscriptions Stated on PS Form 3541 (Include paid distribution above nominal rate, advertiser's proof copies, and exchange copies)	148	134
	(2) Mailed In-County Paid Subscriptions Stated on PS Form 3541 (Include paid distribution above nominal rate, advertiser's proof copies, and exchange copies)	0	0
	(3) Paid Distribution Outside the Mails Including Sales Through Dealers and Carriers, Street Vendors, Counter Sales, and Other Paid Distribution Outside USPS®	30	26
	(4) Paid Distribution by Other Classes of Mail Through the USPS (e.g., First-Class Mail®)	7	5
c. Total Paid Distribution [Sum of 15b (1), (2), (3), and (4)]	▶	185	165
d. Free or Nominal Rate Distribution (By Mail and Outside the Mail)	(1) Free or Nominal Rate Outside-County Copies included on PS Form 3541	3	4
	(2) Free or Nominal Rate In-County Copies Included on PS Form 3541	0	0
	(3) Free or Nominal Rate Copies Mailed at Other Classes Through the USPS (e.g., First-Class Mail)	0	0
	(4) Free or Nominal Rate Distribution Outside the Mail (Carriers or other means)	1	1
e. Total Free or Nominal Rate Distribution (Sum of 15d (1), (2), (3) and (4))	▶	4	5
f. Total Distribution (Sum of 15c and 15e)	▶	189	170
g. Copies not Distributed (See Instructions to Publishers #4 (page 3))	▶	0	0
h. Total (Sum of 15f and g)	▶	189	170
i. Percent Paid (15c divided by 15f times 100)		97.88%	97.06%

* If you are claiming electronic copies, go to line 16 on page 3. If you are not claiming electronic copies, skip to line 17 on page 3.

PS Form **3526**, July 2014 (Page 2 of 4)

16. Electronic Copy Circulation		Average No. Copies Each Issue During Preceding 12 Months	No. Copies of Single Issue Published Nearest to Filing Date
a. Paid Electronic Copies	▶		
b. Total Paid Print Copies (Line 15c) + Paid Electronic Copies (Line 16a)	▶		
c. Total Print Distribution (Line 15f) + Paid Electronic Copies (Line 16a)	▶		
d. Percent Paid (Both Print & Electronic Copies) (16b divided by 16c × 100)	▶		

☒ I certify that 50% of all my distributed copies (electronic and print) are paid above a nominal price.

17. Publication of Statement of Ownership
☒ If the publication is a general publication, publication of this statement is required. Will be printed
in the _____ DECEMBER 2024 _____ issue of this publication.   ☐ Publication not required.

18. Signature and Title of Editor, Publisher, Business Manager, or Owner

Malathi Samayan   Date 9/18/2024

Malathi Samayan - Distribution Controller

I certify that all information furnished on this form is true and complete. I understand that anyone who furnishes false or misleading information on this form or who omits material or information requested on the form may be subject to criminal sanctions (including fines and imprisonment) and/or civil sanctions (including civil penalties).

PS Form **3526**, July 2014 (Page 3 of 4)   PRIVACY NOTICE: See our privacy policy on www.usps.com

Printed and bound by CPI Group (UK) Ltd, Croydon, CR0 4YY

08/05/2025

01864751-0007